YOU CAN

"An honest, humbling, emotional, joyful chronicle of unconditional sibling love. A must-read for parents, teachers and anyone who strives to become a kinder, more compassionate human being."

~ JULIE HANSON, beta reader

"In sharing her truth, Kylainah has shown me a better way to interact with differently abled individuals. I have a new perspective on my own behaviour. Her journey demonstrates growth we can all learn from. Her deep love for her sister shines through the narrative."

~ DEB BROOKS, beta reader

"You Can Find Me in Her Shadow provides a unique glimpse into a world most are unfamiliar with. Zacharczuk's personal, honest, and often raw accounts of her experience of being raised in a family with a special needs sibling have come together as more than a memoir or diary.

Through her words, we, as the greater community, are reminded that not only do we need compassion and understanding for the special needs sibling, but we also need to allow space for the families, parents and siblings to help inform us and guide us as to what their specific needs and supports are throughout their journey. In her first publication, Zacharczuk is providing a voice that few of us hear.

Her observations, and at times, heartbreaking reflections, will resonate for many people living 'in a shadow' while giving hope that others may also find strength in their own voice to access supports they are rightly entitled to.

As educators, medical support, extended family and friends, we need to ask more open-ended questions and provide space for the whole family's needs and support to change as their journey and needs change.

Zacharczuk reminds us that assuming we may know what is best for the sibling of a special needs family, however well intended, can create undo harm that ripples throughout the entire family unit."

~ MICHELLE VAN MANEN, Secondary Special Education Resource Teacher, WSRDSB, beta reader

"As I read your work, I believe that you bring hope, understanding, courage, support and social guidance to everyone who reads and learns your values for human life together."

~MARILYN DALTON, Elementary school teacher, behaviour teacher and mother to 4 children, beta reader

"Captivating! This is a brave and honest recount of the personal struggles of being a sibling to an individual with special needs. I was brought to tears more than once reading about the enduring strain that challenged this young family, and the feelings of loneliness and confusion the author experienced in her younger years. This book shines a light on the often-suppressed emotions and unmet needs of siblings dealing with special needs. This story is important to tell. I highly recommend to anyone experiencing the same challenges in their own journey, and a required read for those supporting special needs families."

~ Chris E, beta reader

YOU CAN FIND ME IN HER SHADOW

MY SISTER HAS SPECIAL NEEDS AND THIS IS MY STORY

Kylainah Zacharczuk

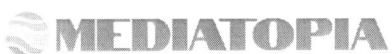

YOU CAN FIND ME IN HER SHADOW

MY SISTER HAS SPECIAL NEEDS AND THIS IS MY STORY

By Kylainah Zacharczuk

First Print Edition 2024

Copyright © 2024 Kylainah Zacharczuk.
All rights reserved.

Cover Photography: Theresa Chalmers
Cover Design: Jeffery Park
Book Design: Dawn Stilwell

Paperback ISBN: 978-1-998290-26-0

No part of this book may be reproduced or used in any manner without written permission from the copyright owner, save for the use of brief quotations in a book review.

DISCLAIMER

Throughout my book, you will notice I use the following words and phrases: special needs, disabled, disability, and differently abled. There could be sensitivity around these terminologies used to describe the special needs community. However, this is the terminology we use in my family.

I respect that your family may choose to use other terminologies which may differ from ours. I have seen and heard other people use the following: person with a disability and/or person with diverse needs, children with diverse abilities, etc.

This is my journey/my story, how it was felt and remembered, and I am not making any claims that what I say throughout this book depicts the lives of all people who live in the spaces of disability.

"Even after all this time, the sun never says to the earth, "You owe me".

Look what happens with a love like that, it lights the whole Sky."

-Hafiz

DEDICATION

For the sibs who feel like they can't relate to their peers. Scared, lost, confused, lonely, and frustrated. The ones who feel they are standing in the depths of their sibling's shadows, reluctant to be seen or heard.

For all those who are in a situation where their loved one is affected by a disability, and find they need to be their voice in the world.

For those who see the differently abled in their communities and truly want to understand their lives and how to interact with them.

For all the parents, grandparents, friends, teachers, doctors, coaches, and within the mental health community, who have someone in their family or know of someone who has a disability, I hope this helps give you clarity and a new view of persons with disabilities and their sometimes-forgotten loved ones.

TABLE OF CONTENTS

Chapter One: Introduction..........Page 1

Chapter Two: What They Didn't Know..........Page 7

Chapter Three: Navigating Life Outside of My Home..........Page 10

Chapter Four: They Won't Let Me Love You-They Are Trying to Keep Us Separated..........Page 18

Chapter Five: I Can't Breathe-They Just Discovered My Secret, I'm Stupid..........Page 25

Chapter Six: You Need Help. You're Not Stupid, You're Just Human..........Page 33

Chapter Seven: A Loving Teacher Who Thought She Could Help..........Page 38

Chapter Eight: It's Not My Sister Creating the Anxiety, It is You..........Page 42

Chapter Nine: Mom Please Don't Have Her Go to High School-Kids Are Mean..........Page 46

Chapter Ten: Who I Am Today..........Page 50

Chapter Eleven: Random Acts of Kindness: Good People Who Wanted to Give My Sister An Experience..........Page 54

Chapter Twelve: Actions Speak Louder Than Words..........Page 58

Chapter Thirteen: What It's Like Being a Sibling of a Special Needs Child..........Page 64

Chapter Fourteen: Trying To Live in the 'Normal' Box..........Page 70

Chapter Fifteen: Lessons from The Shadow..........Page 74

Chapter Sixteen: Stop Asking What Is Wrong with Her!........Page 81

Chapter Seventeen: Stop Staring, It's Rude........................Page 88

Chapter Eighteen: Did That Just Really Happen?..................Page 94

Chapter Nineteen: Dating When You Have a Special Needs Sibling ....Page 103

Chapter Twenty: My Baby Sister..Page 109

Chapter Twenty-One: Dear Baby Sister ....Page 113

Chapter Twenty-Two: Finally Getting My Mother Back......Page 116

Chapter Twenty-Three: She's Not just My Friend, She Is More Like My Sister ....Page 119

Chapter Twenty-Four: You Can Try to Run, But You Can't Hide ....Page 124

Chapter Twenty-Five: Your Parents' Sadness and Fear Is Never Truly Hidden from the SIB; Share It, Explain It, and Heal as a Family (Otherwise, We Both Go through This Alone) 133

Chapter Twenty-Six: My Departing Message to All Those Fellow Special Needs SIBS..Page 136

Acknowledgments: ....Page 140

About the Author: ....Page 142

Resources For the SIBS: ....Page 143

Resources For the Parent: ....Page 146

Index:...Page 148

Where I Found My Research: ....Page 15

PREFACE

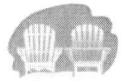

Hi! My name is Kylainah Zacharczuk, and I am the author of the book You Can Find me in her Shadow. My sister has special needs, and this is MY story.

In the beginning, this book was a journal entry, a moment in time I needed to finally remove from my chest. I desperately needed an outlet to finally release some of my childhood traumas, which continued to induce feelings of anxiety for me; the memories and truths that I avoided facing until now.

But the universe has a way of lighting the path you are meant to walk, and so shortly after my first two chapters were on paper, I started bumping into mothers who also had children with special needs. They seemed to be drawn to me, and questions poured from them. They asked if I'd share with them what it felt like for me, being the sibling of a special needs child.

As I listened to them and felt their genuine desire to better understand my perspective, hoping it could inform them on how they could be better parents to their neurotypical children-as they knew their lives were changed as well. I knew it was time to share my story.

And so, my journal writing became a two and a half year, outpour of my deepest thoughts, feelings, insights, and truths. From this, a book emerged; intended to be a resource for others.

As the sibling of a special needs child, few people think of us, our needs, our feelings. I have lived my entire life struggling to fit into this world. Not sure where I'm supposed to plant my feet. One foot in the world of special needs, while the other struggles to blend in with the rest of my peers.

It is my hope that this book may be the bridge that merges these two worlds together, finally.

This book is a story of my life, from my perspective as being the sibling in the special needs space. And while it was extremely difficult to share, I chose to write honestly and allow my authentic truth to speak clearly, knowing that our story might help many other families like ours.

I wrote this book because I personally struggled with knowing how to be a sister to my sibling, and I longed for the resource that might help me.

This book is what I needed. And my mother said that I wrote the book she searched for but couldn't find.

I also wrote this book to shine a light on the community of special needs, to let people see, hear, and understand these people and their families.

And to help the world understand, and recognize in themselves how they intentionally, or unknowingly impact the lives of the person with a disability, and their family.

This book is for parents, to help them understand how much we (the sibling) feel all your emotions, hidden or not, we feel your fear, your guilt, your worry. I write in my book about how its important to not only listen to us, but to include us in the details as much as possible. Be transparent with your child, otherwise we go through this life feeling isolated, confused and alone. Over time, we may master how to hide our feelings, camouflaging them behind a mask of smiles, because we don't want to overwhelm our already stressed family. We might become introverted and scared to raise our hand, afraid that if we don't answer a question correctly, people may assume we have something wrong with us too.

I was personally secretly terrified they'd search for a label for me, like they did my sister. And for years I constantly searched for the disability within my self, not entirely sure how someone gets a disability.

I spent my life, trying to protect my sister from the judgment we felt from the world around us. The constant "What's wrong with her?" "Why can't she talk?" "Why can't she walk?" And sadly, when she finally learned to walk, people would ask, "Why does she walk like that?" and often it was asked right in front of her.

Then, there were the adults who'd asked my parents what is wrong with my sister. After hearing my parents' response, their replies always seemed to be the same, "I'm sorry," after hearing about her disability.

Really! Imagine how my sister felt hearing that. I wanted to be her shield; be her big protective sister, but honestly, I felt helpless.

My sister, and her disability, are embedded into fragments of who I am, how I live in this world, how I see the world, and how I feel it, because of my unconditional love for her.

I would never in a million years trade this life I have with her. I know my sister will never judge me, but instead love me for who I am. Not just because I am her sister, but because of who she is as a person.

She has the kindest soul, and somehow she makes everyone in our lives feel better without being able to speak a single word. Her disability isn't who she is, and I wish the world would look at her the way I do.

In the process of writing this book, I found it not only challenging and stressful, but at times, I even doubted my own abilities to articulate clearly what I had been suppressing for my entire life. I was honestly fearful to share it here with the entire world; my inner most thoughts, feelings, fears, all wrapped and gifted for everyone to experience.

Some of the stories I share within these chapters, I haven't shared with anyone before. Even my parents were hearing them for the first time in the process of writing this book.

My mother wept as I shared my pages with her, each time wiping her tears and expressing to me that, "Parents need to hear this." "I wish I knew this before." "This is important to share."

I witnessed my grandmothers read the first couple chapters of my book, and their reactions were the same; they expressed to me that they hadn't thought about me and my perspective before. They just assumed I was okay and happy.

And then to hear the positive responses from all my beta readers. How they couldn't put the book down, and how they were crying already after only reading the first two chapters.

Someone even shared with me that it inspired her to be a better sibling.

It has been a cathartic experience writing this book, and extremely emotional hearing the beta readers comments that my book was inspiring, informative, and well written.

As I sit here, pen and paper, I find myself wondering, *what does the world need to know?*

The truth is, I've lived my life in two worlds. The world of disability and the world with everyone else. I eventually hid my sister from the world outside that of our special needs community, hoping I could shield her from the truth I was hearing; the actions I was witnessing, the ignorant society that I was struggling to fit into. I thought by concealing my world of special needs from my peers, I'd somehow be protecting my sister. But by doing so, I wasn't living my authentic truth, and because of this, I never felt like I truly belonged anywhere.

As my book came to fruition, and the revisions, and edit process came to an end, an epiphany moment presented itself, and I stared at the possible realization that the sibling may be the bridge.

We stand in the shadows between two worlds that rarely coexist, waiting for them to finally collide and become one. A unity that would finally allow us to take root, as we are the product of both worlds. Yet we navigate this space in secret amongst everyone else, knowing we have been changed by the gifts we've been privileged to receive from our loved ones, and the special needs community.

My hope is that soon, you will, too.

INTRODUCTION

I was five and a half when my baby sister was born, I held her in my arms beside my mother on her hospital bed in admiration. I knew I was going to love, cherish, and protect her forever. However, I was not expecting my life to change so drastically within the years that would follow. Your mother grows a little human inside of her; you anticipate the birth of a healthy, cheerful baby and life afterwards would just continue with another added branch to the family tree.

My little five-year-old self celebrated the fact that I was getting a sibling and better yet, someone with whom I thought I could play with every day. Sadly, it wasn't what I had imagined. I never really had the opportunity to play with my sister the way I knew how to play as a young child. Her arrival came with a lot of challenges and patience that I had not yet discovered during those young stages of my life.

My sister wasn't quite a year old when we were noticing she wasn't following doctors' expectations of the infant-to-toddler development. Life was basically worry, disappointment, sadness, doubt, and fear.

When I was seven years old, my parents were told by the doctors that they were convinced that my sister had a rare disability after struggling to find a diagnosis for her. In order for the doctors to confirm their belief, they needed to run tests. As my parents waited months for these tests to be performed as my sister needed a surgery and genetic testing to confirm this, my parents researched the proposed diagnosis while they waited.

And what they had found terrified them. If the doctors were correct, it meant my sister's time with us on earth would be short lived. The doctors' speculated diagnosis stated that all the children born with this condition died young.

Of course, my parents kept this all hidden from me, or so they thought they did.

On an early Saturday morning, my mother was in the kitchen with a couple of her closest friends, sipping their coffees and chit chatting over a serious topic. I was curious and quite nosey, trying to reach the kitchen without getting seen or heard so I could eavesdrop on their conversation. Then I heard it … was I going to lose my sister?

As I got older, I often questioned myself why I didn't confront my mother about what I had heard in the first place. Maybe I was nervous about getting caught for eavesdropping, or maybe I was really just scared to know the truth.

I contemplated how someone so young could understand this information, or even know how to process these intense and overwhelming emotions.

I didn't understand it; I never wanted this to happen. So, I went up to my sister, slapped her and walked away crying, I remember thinking, how could she do this to me? How could she leave me?

To this day, this memory still lives within me with so much shame and disappointment. I was so frightened and concerned that I was going to live this life without my sister being a part of it, but why would I have shown such unkind and unforgiving behaviour? I realize now I was blaming her when I should have blamed myself.

The truth was, I should have, in that moment, promised her that I would do anything in my power to make sure that she would live the best life possible with the short time we had together. To be the best big sister to her, forever and always. But truthfully, I was scared that I wasn't enough of what she needed me to be. I wasn't strong enough to fight her battles.

Fortunately, all the tests came back negative and as it turns out, my sister does have an extremely rare genetic disorder, but not the devastating diagnosis that the doctors had once predicted. With this new correct diagnosis, we learned God had blessed us with the possibility for a long life with her.

As years passed, we didn't witness my sister's first steps by herself like a neurotypical developing child would have done. My parents left doctor appointments with worry on their faces, and I never heard them talk about their plans and dreams of the day when they become empty nesters and what they'd be doing.

For most people, they would have considered these just normal occurrences; little jabs from mom and dad, "when you kids are gone and out of this house, I am changing your room into a gym. We're going to finally have a little extra money once you're out of the house and on your own, we're going to travel the world." But for our family, this may never happen. As I got older it became clearer to me, like an unspoken truth, my parents didn't talk, celebrate, and maybe never even let themselves dream of a future like the rest of the other parents I knew. We all knew that my sister would always need my parents care for the rest of her life, and that meant for the rest of their lives, too.

I'm sure many families with special needs children would agree that we live our lives in a sea of unknowns. When we plan for the future, we use flexible goals, without holding tightly to an expectation. Because the truth is, whatever the child achieves throughout their life is an achievement within itself and should be celebrated.

So, what was normal? What did a normal life look like? I never understood what that word meant; maybe I thought it was the first years of my younger life.

It was much later as I grew into a young adult, that I understood what the word" normal" meant for me, and I knew my definition was different than my friends'.

It was the first time I became comfortable with the phrase -- this is my truth; this life is my "normal". My family is what keeps me alive, and my sister is the glue that continues to cement this family together.

These special human beings were gifted to our families to teach each one of us about the valuable lessons of love, gratitude, and acceptance, for ourselves and for everything else in this world; to be grateful for what we have, noticing the miracles and the love that life is built on. Others are blinded by the speed and expectations that they have been conditioned to strive towards when building and creating their idea of a "normal life", they don't notice or feel the magnitude of letting go and living an authentic truth- in love, the incredible gift this life gives you. My sister is the reason I understand and value this insight- that was her gift to me.

I love you, my little one who grew up too quickly"

-UNKNOWN

WHAT THEY DIDN'T KNOW

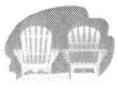

My parents never explained to me about my sister's diagnosis. Nor did they consider that I may need to be guided throughout my childhood about how to communicate her disability with my peers or prep me in knowing how to be a big sister to my sibling who has special needs. The real question is, how would they ever know how to?

What I didn't realize is that we were all trying to figure it out at the same time. Throughout my childhood, we hid a lot from each other about how we were truly feeling and what we were experiencing.

Having good communication between each other and keeping our mental health in check was crucial while learning how to navigate and balance our not-so-predictable life. Most of the time, I thought it would have been easier to just let go of my own thoughts and concerns than let it be a burden to the rest of my family. I didn't want my parents to be consumed with my problems, when they had more than enough of their own. I didn't share how I was feeling or what I was dealing with.

I built habits of even keeping school-related struggles to myself because I didn't want it to be another thing that my parents had to worry about.

I strongly recommend that if you are struggling and feel like you need guidance, don't be like me, ask for help. Even though your parents are attending to your sibling's complex needs, it doesn't mean that they do not want to help you or don't have the time for you.

Once my sister was born, I stopped asking questions, I stopped raising my hand, and I stopped using my voice. I became alone, confused, and angry, escaping to my room, ignoring my parents and even my sister. I started to become less helpful around the house when my father was traveling for work - a time when my mother counted on me the most.

"Education is not the learning of facts, but training the mind to think"

-Albert Einstein

NAVIGATING LIFE OUTSIDE MY HOME

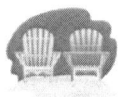

I was raised in a "put yourself in their shoes, people go through way worse things in their lives" type of household. Although, even with this mindset, I didn't know anything about putting my feet in my sister's shoes. In our household, this metaphor meant that I needed to put on her leg braces in order to fully understand what she would have to endure throughout her lifetime, the fear, pain, and restrictions of her daily life.

For the first five years of my sister's life, she would often wake up crying throughout the night. Reflecting on this time, I remember it feeling like forever; like a nightmare that never ended. My bedroom was right beside my sister's, divided by what felt like paper-thin-walls - I could hear everything. Every whimper, every scream, every breakdown. My mother never knew about this, she thought I was fast asleep, dreaming happy dreams.

I remember like it was yesterday, my mother would walk into my sister's room, pick her up, roll her over to her other side, adjust her blankets and if we were lucky, she would fall back to sleep. These events happened several times every night. It was so often that my parents decided to switch their bedroom from their primary suite on the main floor, to the small upstairs guest room right down the hall from my sister and me.

No one knew for sure what prevented her from sleeping soundly but my parents assumed that she might have been experiencing pain because it was so difficult for her to move her body on her own. I always wondered what she felt in those moments of agony.

Have you ever fallen asleep on your arm and when you wake up in the middle of the night and try to move it, your arm feels so heavy that you can barely lift it? No matter how you connect with your arm telling it how to move with your thoughts, you don't have control over it, like it is this dead thing that's attached to your body. It can be scary, and initially in the daze of your awakening, it's a bit confusing.

Now imagine that feeling never going away. Could this have been happening to her entire body because of her lack of ability to move easily throughout the night? At the time, even rolling over and adjusting herself as she slept was impossible for her to do.

Her birth was the start of a long journey of sleepless nights for both my parents and well, unfortunately, for me too. I never expressed to my parents how much this impacted my life until I was much older, and I kept this a secret from both of them. I didn't complain or even mention that her nightly cries kept me up, too. They didn't have a clue that I was struggling like they were. That I laid awake every night, making it a struggle for me to get up the next morning just like it was for them.

As a young child, I never enjoyed the learning part of school as much as being social with my peers. I found myself struggling once my sister was born; it felt like all my parents' attention had been on her. Although, my parents tried their hardest to give me a 'typical' lifestyle as all my friends had lived, we were unintentionally lacking in the educational department.

I remember an event that happened when I was in grade two, at a progress review meeting with my parents and homeroom teacher. They were having a brief discussion about how I was a little behind compared to most of my peers in my class, my teacher quickly brushing it off by saying, "Oh don't worry, this happens a lot with children her age. She will catch up." However, that wasn't exactly what had happened.

Needless to say, both of my parents assumed the teachers would have helped me get caught up and would keep them informed of my progress, guiding them if there was anything they needed to do to support my learning too. But as the years went by, nothing had changed.

It started to feel like because the teachers never took the time to get to know me on a caring and personal level, they didn't know what was going on at home. They didn't know my family was struggling or that I was probably running on a couple hours of sleep each night and my father was usually working away from home, sometimes for months at a time, so it was most often my mother taking care of my sister and me, alone.

In all honesty, I didn't even believe my teachers would have even cared if they knew the truth.

In grade four, I started to skip school a lot. Faking a sickness was common that year for me due to the fact that school started to feel like a burden. Why go somewhere expecting to be a disappointment? I was sad, lonely and missing my father being at home; I was so embarrassed about myself.

My fourth-grade teacher had a lot of heart-breaking events and personal family-related responsibilities, resulting in her having to leave frequently throughout the school year. It felt like she had missed three-quarters of that school year and almost every week we had a new substitute teacher. I didn't want to go to school anymore.

I felt more lost and disappointed in my education than I had ever felt before. I started to believe that maybe I really was stupid, worse yet, I felt like everyone thought so, too. The emotions and stresses I suffered through that year had such a huge impact on me, where it occasionally made me physically ill and I'd call my mother to pull me out of school.

I felt myself introverting that year- losing myself and my friendships in the process.

Within the same year, my sister was awarded the opportunity to attend a special junior kindergarten school classroom at a therapy rehabilitation centre called, KidsAbility. A few times, my mother took me to the centre to volunteer in my sister's classroom- she saw this as a rare opportunity. For me, I saw the chance of volunteering at KidsAbility as not only the distraction I needed at the time, but it felt like a safe place to express who I was. I realized in being there, there were more families just like mine, and it helped me normalize my life in a way I hadn't before.

When I volunteered, I witnessed how the teachers treated my sister; the way they looked at her, loved her, spoke to her and laughed with her. These were special moments with truly good people. I needed to see this and to be around people like them. People who actually understood how to communicate, not only to the child with special needs but also showed me, the sibling, how to be the sibling that my sister would need me to be. They taught me how to communicate with her in a way that I hadn't yet discovered on my own.

I witnessed my parents doing it, but for some reason I needed to witness society accepting her and loving her this way. It was a new perspective, a new way to talk to her and to be okay with accepting nothing in return, maybe just receiving a smile or a hug and sometimes nothing at all. But it never meant that she wasn't listening or that she couldn't understand me.

I began to understand what she was communicating even through her silence. Somehow, I began understanding the jibber jabber, her attempts at speaking the words she was saying in her head. The message was understood in her facial expressions and in her presence - her aura.

Once you let go of the expectations you have - the rules and beliefs we carry about what communication and language looks like, when you quiet yourself, slow down and observe, you become aware and are available to feel and notice the subtle changes in a person's energetic field. You can feel it, you can easily notice all the subtle changes in what they are doing within their body; depending on the person's complex needs, this could be their way of speaking to you.

Like a child before they learn how to speak, they are always attempting to interact with the world around them. It takes practice and patience within yourself to become a skilled observer.

Watching these teachers at my sister's school and witnessing my parents together, opened the door for me to explore within myself how I needed to change and evolve in order to connect fully with my sister and what she was so desperately hoping I'd noticed - she was talking to me, she was answering my questions.

I remember feeling relieved that my sister was attending KidsAbility because she was getting the extra support and love she needed. She was safe and I didn't have to worry about her being there.

My mother knew it was important for me to be around my sister's classmates, who had many complex needs like her own, and these experiences had a enormous impact on my life. This was the first time that I was surrounded by other differently abled children. I got to know them, play with them, my parents invited them and their families over to our house for parties, and I truly connected with them. I will cherish these memories forever; a time where everything just felt normal.

"Sometimes you will
never know the value
of a moment until
it becomes a memory"

-Dr. Suess

THEY WON'T LET ME LOVE YOU – THEY ARE TRYING TO KEEP US SEPARATED

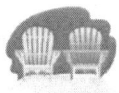

We used to live in a small community, and we were that family that was so different from all the others. Even if there were a few kids with a disability, none were even remotely close to having the severity of complex needs that my sister was born with. At least, that's what I noticed. No wonder why we felt like we couldn't relate to anyone!

I was in grade five when my sister came to my elementary school for her senior year of kindergarten. I remember being so excited to have her there with me. For the first time, she was getting so much attention, and I was so happy to have the opportunity to finally share her with my peers and our small community. Most of the kids from my school knew that I had a sister, but didn't know anything about this part of our life. I kept it all private in hopes to protect her.

This was the opportunity to finally share her with everyone without the awkward conversations of having to explain my sister's rare disability.

I wanted my friends and teachers to see her and get to know her for the incredible human that she is without her complex needs. However, the school was concerned that I needed my own identity, and they tried their hardest to separate the two of us.

When I think back at this time, I felt my duty as the older sibling was not only to protect my sister, but to make sure that she was content within her classroom and that the other kids included her as an equal. That was the only thing that mattered - that her experience being there held good memories for her, and nothing was going to harm her and cause trauma within her life. I was so excited to have her there at my school, and so the first thing my best friend and I did was race to sign up as lunchroom helpers and reading buddies, in hopes we'd be assigned to my sister's classroom as a way to be close to her.

I remember it being so much fun, and I not only found comfort in watching my sister's interaction with her peers and teachers, but I fully enjoyed the experience of being around my sister and the little kids in her class.

I can't exactly recall how much time had passed, I think it was only a couple of months, and then it happened. I was told I wasn't allowed to volunteer in her class anymore. I was devastated! There was no explanation given, no reason why, I was simply told that I was no longer allowed to volunteer in her class. And it felt as though they were preventing me from seeing my sister.

As far as I am aware, no one else had been told that they were no longer allowed to volunteer or that they had to stop.

This caused me a lot of trauma, and I've blocked out a lot of it. I don't even remember who told me or what was said exactly, I just know that I was told I wasn't allowed to go to her class anymore. All I wanted to do was check up on her, even if I had to volunteer over my own lunch breaks to do so.

I was sharing this chapter with my mother, and when I read the part about the teachers trying to separate us by telling me I could no longer volunteer in my sister's class, my mother stopped me in disbelief. She couldn't believe that this had happened to me, and she began sharing with me that my homeroom teacher had called her one day; the memory still vivid in her mind because of how infuriated and disappointed she was with the teacher's request and opinions.

Apparently, my teacher had call to voice her concerns about my behaviours and actions since having my sister in the same school. My teacher was worried that I was putting too much attention on concerning myself with my sister's well being. She felt that it might be interfering with my learning and taking away from my independent identity. The teacher felt I was acting like my sister's caretaker or in other words, acting like my parents, and they strongly felt that it wasn't right for me to take on this parental role.

My teacher explained to my mother that she wanted to prevent me from doing daily pop-ins into my sister's classroom. My mother told her, *"All Kylee has ever wanted was to go to school with her little sister, why couldn't she be allowed to see her?"* Prior to this, I never had many opportunities to share her with my world, my community of peers and teachers. This was my chance to finally be able to share her in hopes that people would love her and see her the way I do!

As a child, all I ever wanted was to be like everyone else, to have the chance to go to school with my sibling, to play together with our friends at the same school. Even the little moments of walking to school and back together each day. In all honesty, I never thought this would be possible. She needed so much extra support, and only certain schools were capable enough to provide it.

I couldn't make sense of why they were moderating my interaction with her. Even if it was for her best interest or maybe for mine, it didn't mean this was handled the right way - the way that considered what my sister would need. After my mother shared this with me, I finally realized why the teachers were trying to prevent me from seeing my sister. But it was only their opinions; it wasn't even the truth.

I wonder if my teachers were even considering my sister's feelings and well-being during these discussions. They didn't even allow enough time for us to be together in the same school, to explore if they were right about their conclusions or just harming us in the process.

As it turned out, I only had one year with my sister. The principal convinced my parents that sending her to another school that specialized in supporting special needs children would provide more support with her learning and skill development.

My family is my sister's eyes, ears, and voice. She can't come home and verbally have a conversation and tell us about her day, what she learnt, what they did, the fun moments she had with her friends, or if someone was mean to her - we wouldn't know. What if the teachers didn't communicate often to my parents, didn't take the time or value the importance of sharing with them? We wouldn't know what was going on throughout her day.

This was why I wanted to be there with her and make it easy to update our family. It wasn't something my parents asked of me, it was just something I wanted to do as the older sibling. Older siblings want to always look out for their younger siblings, to make sure they are safe! My sister is my family and when it comes to family, you look out for one another.

However, my teachers felt that us being there at the same school, was causing "too much stress" on my life. They began to question my memory as my fifth-grade teacher was getting to know me throughout the process of grading my work. She had a false idea of knowing what was right for me and her attempt to try to correct my situation, only did the opposite for me. It affected my relationship with my sister. The teacher was trying to fix a situation that didn't need fixing.

I remember feeling like my teacher wanted me to know that I could trust the adults who were watching my sister, and I needed to believe that she as going to be okay. But I was still a kid, and to me it felt like they were trying to tell me to live a separate life. I was so confused, and because of this, I started to feel embarrassed about my sister, our family and how different we were compared to everyone else. I was now resenting my sister and my parents for having to live this life.

Today, looking back at these moments, I really believe my teacher was likely thinking she was looking out for me; coming from a place of genuinely caring for me and for my future; doing what she thought would be in my best interest. But in this process, she entirely avoided acknowledging my sister's well-being.

Although, my teachers wouldn't allow me to volunteer anymore, no one stopped me from popping in to check up on her once in a while, but I eventually stopped going to my sister's class altogether and I don't exactly remember why. All I remember was that because I had stopped going to her classroom, it seemed like my teacher was happy. Looking back, she likely thought I was stepping out on my own and it would be good for me but it wasn't.

During the remainder of the school year, my mother later found out that I went to my sister's classroom less frequently, and eventually, I stopped altogether. I never told my mother when or why I had stopped going to see her - the teachers told her. My mother thought I didn't want to go see her, that I stopped entirely on my own because I didn't care about her being there anymore, and I didn't tell her any differently.

"In the end, some of your greatest pains, become your greatest strengths."

-Drew Barrymore

I CAN'T BREATHE – THEY JUST DISCOVERED MY SECRET. I'M STUPID

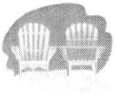

When I got my first report card in the mail during my fifth grade of elementary school, I was sitting at the kitchen table going through the contents with my mother by my side. Some of my grades were so low that she called my teacher immediately to ask what was going on.

My mom was furious! At the time, I wasn't sure if she was mad at my teacher for giving me these poor grades or if she was really just disappointed with me. I remember her asking the teacher, how is it that I am in grade five and she's now just finding out how far behind I was in my learning! My teacher returned with a reply, "You know, sometimes when the child is stressed, they tend to forget. Teachers sometimes forget, too." But how can you do that, unless you really aren't concerned about my education!

I remember my mother saying if only she knew about this earlier, she could've helped me catch up, to get me back on track with the rest of my peers. None of my previous report cards from any of my grades prior to then had reflected this level of trouble I was having in some of my subjects. Other than my second-grade teacher, none of my former teachers had expressed to my parents their concerns about my continued struggles. None of my report cards reflected a student that should have been failing.

After these difficult conversations with my mother, my homeroom teacher advocated for the support I needed so I could receive access to the qualified staff who assessed students. Their job is to determine where the student is currently at in their learning, and to also help create a detailed plan for the teachers which included resources and guidelines on what was needed in order to support the student

This information from this assessment would provide my teacher with instructions, support and what she would need in order to understand how to teach me; essentially identifying my learning style and finding the holes I had in my learning from the previous years.

A meeting was held between my mother, my homeroom teacher and the support teacher to discuss my case.

In research for writing this book, my mother and I spoke about this conversation, where the support teacher verbalized her opinion that I see a psychologist for testing. She suggested I get a Psychoeducational Assessment first before they went any further.

I can only imagine my mother's irritation at this moment. Knowing her, she likely stared at this woman like she had two heads and ten eyeballs!

"Why would we need this done? We have more than enough information to come up with a plan that is needed in order to help her," my mother spoke.

My teacher backed her up in agreement. "I have all the information that I would need to support the fact that she requires this additional support".

After which the support teacher added, "Some parents feel like they would like to have an answer as to why their child is struggling. Most of them felt like it was helpful for them to have a label, a reason why".

My mother looked at the lady in utter disbelief and said, "Our family has had enough labels, she will not be tested. You have enough information that we have provided to determine the fact that she needs extra support in order for you to access the funding you need to see this through".

Finally, the support teacher looked at my homeroom teacher and they both agreed in unison, "Okay, we will move forward then".

That summer, my mother decided to make sure we were supporting my education. This included working on the subject I disliked the most, math! It's a subject that builds like a tower of blocks, one on top of the other. You need to understand each step fully before adding another. Without this foundational grasp of the subject, your tower won't scale very high, and you will find yourself with a pile of blocks on the floor with no clue what they are and what to do with them. This is how it had always felt for me.

I found math very challenging and most often would try running away from the subject. The truth was, no matter how many attempts I gave, the information went through one ear and out the other. Every time I thought I understood it, I actually had the answer wrong, I couldn't make sense of why I wasn't grasping the subject. I had gotten my hopes up with the idea that I was understanding it, just to get disappointed. I started to believe I truly was stupid; how could I have been so naive to think I was getting it right when I was in fact always getting the answer wrong.

My mother wanted to help me fill in the holes that I was missing. This meant working on my math everyday for the entire summer going into the sixth grade.

Initially, I was resisting doing it and I wasn't prepared to put in the work it required of me, especially over my summer break and within the short amount of time we had to catch up. The last thing I wanted to do on my time off was more school, more of the subject that I loathed the most, the thing that made me feel so small, useless, and ashamed.

My mother recognized my resistance for what it was: embarrassment, guilt, fear, and hopelessness. All the stories I believed of myself at the time- the reasons I couldn't understand school like everyone else. These thoughts continued to play in my head, and I was trying to run away from them like I would a storm of bullies trying to catch me.

My mother gently sat beside me, looked me in the eyes and with conviction said to me, "Kylee, this isn't your fault, this is my fault, this is the teachers' fault. You are not stupid. We are going to get through this and help you get caught up. But I need you to know, you are not dumb. We're going to work on this, but this is now the time to put in real effort and attention. You can't run away from this anymore".

The truth was, no matter how many times my mother tried to reassure me throughout this process that it wasn't my fault and that I wasn't an idiot, I still didn't believe her. I thought it was always going to be my truth; it didn't matter or change my belief that I had of myself.

At this point, I thought I was not capable of being intelligent- that it wasn't even possible for me to catch up. I was terrified that there was something wrong with me. I was afraid that I had a disability too, like my sister.

But of course, that wasn't the truth, it was that mob of bullies in my head convincing me, petrifying me into a state of chronic fear and eventually, a paralyzing hopelessness due to this false truth that I had made up of myself.

That September, after a long summer of learning math, my mother contacted the support teacher and asked that I be re-tested before the new school year began. He was reluctant, saying it was typically not protocol to retest at this time. He also stated that, "Often they notice that the students actually regress slightly over the summer break".

The determined mother that I have, after this discussion, advocated strongly and refused to take no for an answer, knowing how hard we had worked and witnessing the changes within me and my understanding of the subject.

To my teacher's surprise, I not only exceeded all of his expectations, but he said to my mother that in all of his years teaching, he's never seen a student advance so quickly.

I was a classic case of a kid who needed an intervention so much sooner and as I write this chapter today, I can't help but wonder why nobody jumped in sooner to save me.

Was it because they didn't want to upset my family or put more on my parents' plate?

Maybe they didn't want to put in the work because they saw me as a huge project that they didn't have the time for, so they just closed their eyes and waited for the next teacher to take over? It felt like they had given up on me. Sometimes, I felt like they were mad at me because my grades were so low that it would ultimately make them look like they are bad at their job. So instead, they let me stay behind just like an abandoned puppy that no one wants to put in the work to take care of.

Or worse, did they just assume I likely had a learning disability just like my sister? Did they think there was nothing they could do to help me? Or they didn't want to be the person who had to inform my parents about their assumptions. Did they even worry about me?

The problem was, I was scared my fears would become my reality, that one day they'd tell me something was wrong with me, too. As sad as it was, I witnessed how being around people with special needs changed how my peers would act. They didn't know how to relate to them, and because of this they created distance between them and the differently abled person. I was scared that they would do the same with me if they knew I was struggling and possibly had a learning disability. These thoughts would constantly swarm in my brain on a daily basis. I saw the changes in people, and right away a normal issue of needing extra help understanding something, caused me immediately to feel shame and fear as I questioned, "What is wrong with me?" I automatically assumed that people would judge me, or that someone would find something different about me.

I don't think someone growing up in a typical household would normally think this way about themselves. Because of my family's situation, I think I have spent my entire life running away from anything I felt was hard, out of fear that one day someone would tell me that my fate is the same as my sister's. I know how difficult and alone that road is.

"Maybe the journey isn't so much about becoming anything.

Maybe it's about un-becoming everything that isn't really you so you can become who you were meant to be in the first place."

www.dreamsforbreakfast.com

YOU NEED HELP. YOU'RE NOT STUPID, YOU'RE JUST HUMAN

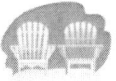

There are multiple reasons why someone might be struggling with learning. It doesn't have to mean you have a disability or a permanent learning difficulty, and it definitely doesn't mean that you have a genetically predetermined likelihood that you have a disability like your sibling.

For most of my childhood, I found myself trapped in dark thoughts, worried if I found something difficult to understand, it could mean I had a disability too. No one explained to me what disability was or how it happens. There were so many questions around understanding why someone had a disability and others don't. I found myself looking for the disability within myself, not understanding the difference between finding a subject difficult and actually having a learning disability. So, I hid everything in hopes it would disappear, and no one would know the truth.

Schools need to consider the effects of the language they choose to use with parents and the sibs of special needs families when communicating.

In families with special needs children, life is overwhelming, and labels highlight to us that the world thinks we don't belong. It can feel sad, embarrassing, painful and for the sibling hearing that someone is looking for their label too now, it is devastating. They know what the label means; it means that they are different from their peers, and they know that if they receive a label, the world will look at them like something is wrong with them too.

I wish everyone thought about my needs and supported me differently. I feel that when supporting the sibling who may be showing signs of struggling to learn, the first step should never be to look for a label. The first step should be supporting the sibling and their family's mental health. Chronic stress can affect the brain and body. It can lead to brain fog, poor short-term memory, lack of focus and concentration, and so much more. The school should be supporting the sibling by recommending that the family seek counselling from a therapist experienced in working with families with disability; supporting their mental health as they navigate their world of special needs. The school should recommend the family seek support and guidance from their family doctor or Naturopathic doctor to resolve any hormonal imbalances effecting the body and brain due to the chronic stress that they have likely been drowning in.

Additionally, they may find benefit by adding Biofeedback and Neurofeedback as these are techniques that have been known to calm the nervous system. And ABM® NeuroMovement®, "wakes up the brain to create new connections and new patterns that dramatically improve physical, cognitive, and emotional performance."

After which, if this doesn't improve the child's ability to learn and concentrate at school, then at that time, a Psychoeducational Assessment by a psychologist should be done to determine the underlying reason for the sibling's continued learning difficulty.

This is a much gentler way to approach this situation that allows the sibling to feel supported and heard without the attention or assumption that something could be genetically wrong with them. They will feel normal, realizing that their difficulties are valid within the circumstances that they have been living in, and the learning struggles that they have been experiencing can be resolved.

According to Bruce Lipton, PhD, stem-cell biologist and author of *The Biology of Belief,* the subconscious mind is programmed between the ages of zero to seven. This means that during this time frame, your strongest beliefs of the world are formed. They are your core beliefs, values, cheerleaders, and unfortunately, your inner bullies. You take in what people say around you, what they feel or what they believe is true.

I wonder if I had help earlier, if I would have had a much smaller group of bullies banging on the closed doors in my mind.

In moments that cause stress for me such as, taking a test, speaking in front of a very large crowd, and even writing this book - sharing my most personal, private and innermost thoughts (some of which I had never shared with my own parents until now) I am constantly consumed with anxiety; fearing I will fail, be judged, or will find myself being ignored.

In the process of writing my story, I found myself facing moments where I hadn't spent enough time addressing those fears, the part of my subconscious programming that tells me I'm a failure, so I don't even try; that I'll get hurt, broken and that most likely no one cares how I am. These are the constant thoughts and fears that are in my head as I bravely attempt to share myself with the world around me.

Maybe, just maybe, if my stress and fears were addressed earlier on, that gang of tormenting meanies in my mind, instead might be one lonely jerk who annoyingly pipes up with some BS comment and then is quickly shut down by the roaring cheers; an encouraging entourage who always has my back, following me around and never leaves my side. Most importantly, they never allow me to give up on anything I want to try.

Today, I still struggle, trying to quiet the sound of the banging bullies that stand at my sealed tight door that I closed off within the contents of my brain. I learned through practice, focusing on the images in my mind of my mother's loving face, my sister's cheerful smile, and I imagine my dad's comforting hugs as they all cheer me on. I use them as a reminder to myself, that I've got this, and failing only exists if I don't try- and what's the fun in that!

*"Let yourself cry.
Let yourself feel frustrated
And angry. Let yourself
feel the pain but know that
it's going to pass."*

-Emma Chamberlain

A LOVING TEACHER WHO THOUGHT SHE COULD HELP

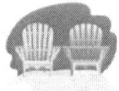

I knew my fifth-grade teacher cared deeply for me, and I truly appreciated her continued support and honesty. For the first time, I felt heard and seen in my own classroom.

She never criticized or made me feel small for not understanding. She was the first person to lead my family in discussions about the extent to which my grades didn't comply to the educational standards.

But it wasn't until I became a young adult, as I reflected back on these profound moments and listening to my mother's version of what was happening to me during this period. The conversations that were being discussed behind my back about me that she had with the school- all of which I wasn't even aware of, I realized how detrimental it was to my relationship with my sister, my parents, and with myself. It increased my overwhelming fears of being different because of my sister. I was terrified that the world would judge me and my family.

My teacher didn't come from the world of special needs- the world that my family lives in. This is a different arena that plays by different rules. What she didn't consider was that there's no hiding when it comes to family; it doesn't matter that my sister has a disability or not, she is who she is. She and her disability are embedded into fragments of who I am, how I live in this world, how I see the world and how I feel it because of my unconditional love for her. She's my sister, I love her.

Yet somehow during this time, my sister was put into a different kind of box. My teacher went behind my mother's back, thinking she knew better. She made assumptions that my sister was the cause of all my learning difficulties, and she thought my stress would be reduced by living a separate life from hers - but this was my life!

I felt persuaded to worry less about my sister, and to view her as my parents' responsibility.

Even after my parents said, no, that they didn't want us separated, that they wanted me to be able to see her, I was somehow coerced to leave her behind.

The thing that really saddens me today was that I really liked this teacher. She was kind to me. She showed me compassion and love more than any teacher had before. She was always there for me, waiting with an open hand and at the time, I really did need it. I knew she wanted to help me and support me. Still to this day, I have so much appreciation for her, for shining a light on me. But what she did changed the course of the rest of my life growing up. It turned me into a person I didn't want to become - it messed up my identity. It wasn't fair for my sister, and it caused a lot of disconnect within my relationship with her, within myself, with my parents, and how I interacted with others. I was trying to live a lie, a different version of myself, one from a different reality.

Now that I am older, reflecting back on this situation and looking at the events of my life, what I have gone through and how I have felt living this life – I feel that where my teacher missed the mark was that instead of separating me and my sister, I needed guidance on how to merge my two worlds in a harmonious way.

If you are a teacher, a coach, a community member, an extended family member or family friend - anyone who has an influence with the sibling within the special needs family, be very careful and mindful with your words, your intentions, and with sharing your own beliefs based on your experiences when communicating to the sibling. You may feel like you are supporting them and guiding them, but know that the child with special needs is never a problem and should never be expressed that they are one. They are unique and loved. And together as a unit, the family navigates this world differently than you can ever imagine or relate to.

"Leaves don't cling onto the branches of a tree. They fall off and create new leaves. It's the same as breaking ties with the past and creating new possibilities and experiences."

-Anonymous

IT'S NOT MY SISTER CREATING THE ANXIETY, IT IS YOU

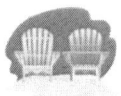

The school arranged a practice fire drill; this was going to be my sister's first time ever hearing the roaring alarms, the teachers shouting as they instructed the children to stand into single file lines outside on the school's premises.

My classroom hustled through the double exit doors following the lead of my teacher. I remember feeling really anxious, wondering how my sister was doing as she was experiencing this for the first time. I wanted to check up on her to make sure she was okay. I thought if she had me next to her, it would help comfort her and get her through all the loud chaos without her feeling terrified as she normally does with loud unexpected noise.

So, I summoned the courage to ask my teacher if I could go see her to make sure she wasn't freaking out. But she brushed me off angrily and spoke, "No, you can't! She will be fine. The teachers are already helping her, they're there with her. You need to go back to the end of the line." I stood there in utter disbelief; did she really just say that to me?

In my head I questioned, how would you know, you haven't even met my sister, you don't know her. I understood that it was a fire drill, but I witnessed other students lining up with other classes and I knew that the teachers were marking them down as an extra in their line. How fair was it that they could, but I wasn't allowed?

My teacher thought that my sister was my problem, that she was giving me anxiety. But really, it was my teacher that was creating extreme anxiety for me by preventing me from seeing my sister in a situation where I knew this was likely traumatic for her.

She didn't let me protect her like a big sibling would. I remember thinking, "*I just want her to know that she was going to be okay. That she was safe, she didn't have to worry, and I was there for her. Why won't they let me help her when I know she was probably scared and would feel safer with me.*"

The stress continued...

Even all those times when I was called down to the principal's office, only to be told that my sister had gotten picked up and brought home by my parents. I remember pleading with them to give me an explanation as to why she was gone, but the teachers wouldn't budge.

I remember one time in particular, I could tell on their faces that they were worried about my sister, and that escalated my fears even more. They sucked at hiding their nervous facial expressions.

Again, I sat alone and questioned, why wouldn't they tell me? Not receiving an answer was driving me insane; did something bad happen to my sister and they couldn't tell me?

For the rest of the school day, it was all I could think of - distracted in my thoughts, thinking the worst possible things imaginable. After the last bell rang, I ran home as quickly as I could to find out that my sister had multiple seizures that morning.

However, since writing this book, my mother told me that she remembers this day. The teacher and secretaries at the front office asked her if they should tell me what had happened and why my sister had to leave school early. It was my mom who said no. She thought it was best to tell me herself once I came back home from school.

But the truth was, it was important for me to have better communication and transparency about this situation, instead of all of them trying to hide their horrible poker faces so they wouldn't worry me.

Hiding it from me made me more stressed, filling me with so much anxiety from fearing the worst. They all should have involved me, helping me to understand and learn how to adjust to my sister's unknowns; our families ongoing roller coaster ride taking us on a journey to places most people never go or experience, at least in my small world.

"Nothing ever goes away

until it teaches us what

we need to know."

-Pema Chodron

MOM PLEASE DON'T HAVE HER GO TO HIGH SCHOOL - KIDS ARE MEAN

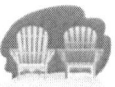

I remember the last bell ringing at the end of the school day, the buses waiting outside to bring us home, the kids crowded in the long, narrow hallways, rummaging around pulling their bags from out of their lockers.

Students departed out of the automatic doors at the end of the hallway at the same time as other students emerged out of the classrooms on either side of the exit, making it feel claustrophobic with the potential risk of getting run over or bumped in the head with a backpack or an elbow, especially if you were me - who is five feet tall.

The special needs classroom was located next to these exit doors - two rooms down to be exact, however instead of safely escorting these students to their buses before the other students, they were exiting their classrooms at the same time as the crowd of arrogant people who rushed down the hall and burst out the school like a stampede of bulls, careless and unapologetic.

On this particular day, I was trying to get past a group of tenth graders in front of me. They were walking so slowly; it was testing my patience. I was close to missing my bus, and so at this point I had no choice but to run past them, then I heard it

They were making fun of the younger, differently abled teenager when they saw him in the hallway, as he was standing outside his locker packing up his bags. Spoken a little quieter on purpose, but loud enough that I could hear every single word, they commented how they were frightened of him, "He looks weird," they said. "He doesn't look normal." And they all laughed and agreed in unison.

I don't even remember who these guys were and that doesn't matter, what I do remember was how they were making fun of an innocent young man who had special needs- they portrayed him as a circus freak.

They looked at him like he was an alien in our school who was so strange and so different from everyone else- he was peculiar in their arrogant eyes.

I felt terrible for him; a wave of sadness washed over me- for my sister, for this kid, and for anyone else who experiences this. All I wanted to do was help him, protect him from this cruel world. But I didn't know how.

How was I supposed to change these boys' perspectives? How was I supposed to explain it to them? Even if I spoke about my opinion of what they had said, would it have made such an impact on them? Was it possible that they would never speak so low about someone who is differently abled again or anyone else for that matter?

It was at this moment I vowed that my sister was never going to my high school, I had so much fear for her going to any normal high school, period.

I remember confronting my mom, persuading her to not let my sister go to high school.

"Mom, please don't send Mikaela to my high school. I can't protect her there. I'm five years older, I won't even be there when she is old enough to go, please listen!"

"The future depends

on what you

do today."

-Mahatma Gandhi

WHO I AM TODAY

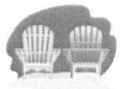

At the age of fifteen, my family moved and traveled across the United States for the next three years of my life. The first year, I slipped into a deep depression as I lost all my friends, and my worst fears had now become my reality - I was now completely alone.

But I realized that without these experiences, and at times difficult emotions that I went through, I never would have transformed into the person that I am today.

I was finally starting to focus on myself and strengthening the relationships between me and my family.

I was no longer consumed with my old beliefs and expectations, thinking we needed to be this picture-perfect family. I wasn't striving to be the person I thought society expected me to be in order to fit in anymore. I no longer worried about answering people's questions about my sister. I was so consumed with my assumptions and past beliefs of who I needed to be in society, that I knew it was time that I let them go. They weren't serving me; in fact, they were destroying me. It felt like it was literally poison in my body.

And in that moment of epiphany, I had of myself, and of my family, I had a new sense of relief; like a million waves had washed over me, removing every heavy and negative layer I had been holding onto which had been slowly drowning me. In that moment, I chose to believe that nothing was going to bring me down anymore. Those old opinions no longer holding power, preventing me from being my authentic self. A person who *proudly* stood by my sister.

I had begun this new phase in my life where nothing else mattered in the world except for my family. Our family's distance from our old life was what we all needed; an unexpected journey where we laughed together and ultimately healed together.

Through the process of writing this book, I had a deep discussion with my parents about how on this journey, something so magical had taken place. That even though we had our struggles while living in hotel rooms and as we traveled crammed together, spending every hour of the day together, we ended up creating this inseparable bond. For the first time, I had a chance to build a strong relationship with my sister and with my parents. I let down my wall, I showed them who I was, and I learned more about them than I had ever before.

As my family healed together, we grounded as a unit, no matter what comment came our way, or eyes we saw staring over at us, even the arrogant opinions from either friends, family members, or strangers that were expressed, it could not break us anymore. Our connection, love, and devotion for each other was more powerful than their words, and we wouldn't let it affect us like it once had.

My sister contributes so much love, compassion, and warmth to our lives, truly making our family whole. If you would have told me earlier that my family would explore different states and experience the coolest tourist attractions together as a whole family, I'm not sure if I would have believed you.

Even though at times traveling didn't go as planned, there were concerns for my sister's safety and if we couldn't do something together, it was because it wasn't accessible for her. Sometimes there were situations were only two of the four of us would be able to experience a place or event. In those moments, we did find ourselves reminded of the difficulty and unfairness of my sister's disability; circumstances where it prevented us from experiencing things as a whole family.

"The best and most beautiful things in the world cannot be seen or even touched, they must be felt with the heart."

-Helen Keller

RANDOM ACTS OF KINDNESS: GOOD PEOPLE WHO WANTED TO GIVE MY SISTER AN EXPERIENCE

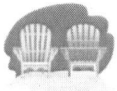

Salt Lake City, Utah Airport

During a flight to San Fransisco, California for Neuromovement® lessons for my sister at the Anat Baniel Method clinic, we arrived in Salt Lake City airport waiting for our connecting flight. As we patiently waited in our terminal for our second plane to arrive, we ended up having an encounter with a Delta employee who was checking us onto our flight.

He looked at my sister, then at my mother and so kindly asked if we wanted to follow him onto the airplane so my sister could experience sitting up in the cockpit of the plane and meeting the captain!

He even upgraded our tickets to better seats on that flight, so it made it easier for my mother and I to get my sister off the plane safely once we had landed.

Off to the Grand Canyon

We drove from Fort Worth, Texas to San Fransisco, California. Deciding to take in the sites on the way to our destination, the Grand Canyon was on the top of our list.

We were driving down the zigzagged mountain roads of Arizona with our windows down, the cool wind whipping through our open windows. My sister's wheelchair parking pass tucked away between the seats, and without us realizing what was about to happen, the wind blew the parking pass straight out of the window, lost on the cliff of that mountain road. With no safe place to pull over or turn around, the parking pass was gone forever.

For the rest of the drive both my parents sat in silence, hesitant for our arrival, wondering how far we might have to walk with my sister to witness one of the most breath-taking views that we had all been dying to experience. Most importantly, they worried how much my sister could handle or tolerate since we wouldn't be able to park in an accessible parking spot without a parking pass.

When we arrived at the park, to our surprise, the park ranger gave us a full day pass to drive through the gated roads, this meant that we could drive around the Grand Canyon rather than walk to see the view.

The Private Viewing of the Baby Animals

The manager at a small city zoo had given my sister and our family a full private tour of their zoo and even a special opportunity to view and pet many of the baby animals that were enclosed there. Each of these animal encounters were probably a once-in-a-lifetime experience, and because of my sister, I was able to experience this rare opportunity too.

Prior to visiting the zoo, my mother called and explained about my sister and her situation, she then proceeded to ask if their zoo offered closer and intimate interactions with any of the smaller animals. The zoo organizer confirmed that they would do something better. They had a daily show where they showcased some of the baby animals born at the zoo for all the children to see up close.

If it weren't for these kind-hearted people, my sister would not have ever experienced these extraordinary opportunities which brought so much joy to both of us. I hoped that they noticed her glowing smile on her beautiful face, and that they knew that what they did for her was all worth it. That they knew how truly appreciative we were as a family. My hope is that one day more people will be like them, and that we'd live in a benevolent society.

"When thinking about life,
remember this:
No amount of guilt
can change the past,
and no amount of
anxiety can change
the future."

-Unknown

ACTIONS SPEAK LOUDER THAN WORDS

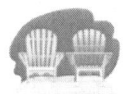

It has been my experience that in today's society, many continue to view the special needs community through the lens of generations past. Where not so long ago, this community was victim to a society that viewed them through prejudicial eyes, allowing for sinister acts of abuse and cruelty to this vulnerable, loving, and innocent community.

Generations of fogged perceptions filled with misunderstanding and ignorance, seem to continue to plague the lives for people with disabilities.

A community of people who may find it difficult to speak easily for themselves and who are cared by families who have, for generations, tried their best to protect and shield them from a world who saw them through a broken lens. A world who thought disability rendered a person broken, faulty, or worse.

I don't understand how this is still going on today, at a time when we are in a culture where people value the importance of breaking free of societal norms, and the powers that willed society to stay in the boundaries of acceptable beliefs systems are shifting.

But yet, society is still not shining a light on the importance of embracing this community.

You may think you are not judgmental, that you don't discriminate against the special needs community. Maybe you don't partake in making jokes about a person's disability, you might even believe you hold compassion for them and wish them and their family well.

You may not believe that you have an aversion towards a disabled person, and you may not think that you discriminate them. But how do you think they feel when you talk above them to their caregivers instead of talking directly to them? Do you talk to everyone else in the room except for the person with special needs?

Do you catch yourself staring at them? Do you say hello? Or do you choose to talk to everyone else around them and completely ignore them like they aren't even there. Are you guilty of not including them? Not embracing them like you would do with everyone else.

If this sounds like you, then the real question is, are you uncomfortable or are you really just ignorant?

I've had people admit to me, that they don't know how to act around people who have special needs because it makes them feel uncomfortable about themselves.

They have shared with me that they find it hard to know how to communicate to someone who is non-verbal when explaining to me how they feel around my sister. It has been difficult for me to grasp how someone else's difficulty can alter a person's ability to communicate. Once they shared this confession with me, I remembered looking at them with a bit of shock and I questioned them, do you find it hard to connect with a young child who is not yet speaking? You don't, do you? You connect with them and communicate with them following their non-verbal cues. It's the same thing!

You connect to them with kindness, you treat them with dignity, respect, and with inclusion. You let them know that they are valued like you would with anyone else - this is how you treat a person who has special needs.

Have you ever excluded a differently abled person from your plans because you can't imagine how they could participate? Or worse, you assumed they wouldn't know the difference if they were left out of your fun. Do you let them watch from the side lines? Or choose to not invite them at all.

These exclusions hurt them, and it alienates them and their family. Your ignorance makes them feel like they are not important and that no one cares about them.

They feel like they're invisible, unwanted and alone.

I've witnessed this happen to my sister her whole life, and it's heartbreaking.

Imagine someone walking into a room with everyone you know, the person smiles and says hello to everyone except for you. They completely ignore you, looking past you as they scan the room. Maybe your friends and family are in this room, and this person talks to them but pretends like you weren't even there. Or worse, maybe this person is one of your family members or family friends, and yet they still ignore you like you don't belong there. They may even sit at the table and make conversations with everyone else but you.

How would you feel to have people not want to take the time to make a real connection with you? Not even make eye contact with you. Does being ignored feel good? Do you feel worthless? Do you feel invisible yet?

Just because someone can't speak back to you the way you are used to, it doesn't mean that they don't feel or understand you. It's possible they are speaking what they want to say in their head, and their ability to organize their thoughts into verbal spoken words isn't available for them. But this doesn't mean that they don't understand and don't want to be included.

Everyone wants to feel valued, we want to be heard, and people want to be loved and accepted for who they truly are.

Everyone feels energy, everyone wants to feel important, even if from the surface it doesn't look that way.

Today's society speaks strongly and passionately for power of choice and freedom to express who they are without judgment. They continue to demand this from the world, knowing that it should be our human right to not be judged, discriminated or excluded because of who you are.

Like these activists, these visionaries and power houses leading and empowering this movement of equality, you, too, can support this much needed change. True social evolution will only take place when we fully embrace and view each other with kindness, respect, and inclusion for all walks of life.

Disability is a part of every race, every culture, and religion in every corner on this planet.

We need to stop ignoring this community! I think you are lucky if you get to know these souls; they will bless your life with so much love, and you will gain wisdom only an open-heart experiences through the teachings of empathy.

I am so grateful that my sister is alive and that she is in my life, my internal light shines brighter because of her.

"I don't forgive people because I'm weak, I forgive them because I am strong enough to know people make mistakes."

-Marilyn Monroe

WHAT IT'S LIKE BEING THE SIBLING OF A SPECIAL NEEDS CHILD

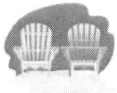

If you are a sibling of a special needs child, I want you to know that it's okay to let yourself feel the emotions that we have about our complicated life. Maybe you relate to me and have gone through and have dealt with similar thoughts and concerns, and maybe you've had similar reactions as I have had. What we have to remind ourselves is to notice what triggers these emotions and fears, accepting them for what they are.

Bring forth your questions as to why you are feeling the way you are. I want you to know that we are all on this journey together and most importantly, know you are definitely not going to be alone through it, even if you feel this way at this present moment.

It may feel disappointing at times, even a bit confusing, frustrating, or embarrassing, but I promise you, you will realize that the life we live now is a privilege and we need to honour it for all that it is. You may be questioning what I mean by this. Well, it's simple. Our siblings are true gifts, and we are the lucky ones having them a part of our families. Throughout every year they teach us so many valuable things that we aren't even aware of.

It doesn't matter if you are the older sibling or even the younger sibling, we are held with a lot of responsibilities and expectations even at a young age. Because of this, we tend to grow up a lot faster than our peers, making it sometimes extremely difficult to relate to most people.

Your obligations and duties as the sibling are so not comparable to your friends'. At times, this can be so challenging; the relationship between you and your special needs sibling is often different than if you were to compare it to other typical sibling relationships. We had to mature, and in a way, we had to provide a space where our sibling was able to be put first, their needs above our own.

As the sibling, we are more observant, cautious, and more aware of others' feelings and emotions because our siblings teach us how to feel. We can see what our sibling goes through every day of their life; the pain, the anger, the disappointment, the happy moments and the times of comfort and peace. Our siblings teach us to become in-tuned within ourselves so we can understand what they go through, and we find ourselves evolving and changing in the process. We generously put our siblings before ourselves because we know they need to be.

It's kind of ironic that once our siblings are born into this world, we end up forgetting what life was like before them. As I grew older, it became harder and harder to relate to my peers and their families. It seemed like there were very few families that were similar to mine, making it feel like it was impossible for us to align our lives together, almost like we were on two different planets spinning in opposite directions. And even if I had found siblings with lives like mine, I found it very difficult to grow friendships with them. There always seemed to be a huge age gap between us; everyone was so much younger or so much older.

A journey filled with so many ups and downs, moments of complete happiness to moments of total grief and despair. Maybe they haven't yet had the same discoveries as I had; what it means to be the sibling. Sometimes I worried that I was running away from having these opportunities of making friends with other siblings because I didn't want to relate to people like me or confront what my family goes through. But we live a very interesting life that makes us, us. Our siblings will be the one person in our lives that will always be there for us on the sunny days and on the dark ones, no matter what we look like or what we accomplish, they love us.

Growing up, I can only recall three other families in my old hometown who had a family similar to mine, but although the siblings were only a little older than me, we were never close. At the time I wondered, had I been more comfortable with the whole underlying concept of what special needs meant to me, would I have been able to nurture a relationship with them? Maybe we both would have learned from one another, looked out for each other, receiving guidance that I so badly needed. I was worried that because they were older than me, they wouldn't want to hangout with someone younger. But looking back, I wonder if maybe they were trying to protect me, because I know I did that with other families with younger siblings. Or maybe they just didn't want to talk about it and perhaps they were going through the process of navigating their own life; the life of being the sibling of a special needs child.

The truth was, we were all still learning, growing, and developing on our own separate paths. Maybe we weren't ready to give advice to each other because we hadn't yet healed our own wounds enough to be available to be someone else's support system.

Most of the hard times are hidden beneath camouflaged smiles, so others don't realize how exhausted and broken we are. We hide our emotions as a shield to help keep a positive attitude for our sibling and for our parents. I concealed my loneliness, my anxieties and my fears hidden behind the shadow of my smile; I forced these feelings into the darkest places of myself so that no one could see.

I thought I didn't want to show how weak I felt, but deep down I didn't know how to feel anymore. Almost like I was being sucked into my own emotions but too scared to voice how I truly felt, and I didn't want to be the cause of everyone's problems.

Thankfully, I've grown to disagree with this belief system. We need to voice up! I have written this book to not only inspire you, but I'm here to be your friend so you know you're not alone. When you feel like no one understands you or relates to what you are going through, know I understand you. I love you; I appreciate you, and you are being heard. I want you to know that you are doing a good job and that I am *so* proud of you and how far you have come today. Your life is just beginning.

"If you want other people to accept your sibling, the first one that needs to accept your sibling is yourself."

-Chaya Wertman (YouTube video: Resources for Teen Siblings)

TRYING TO LIVE IN THE 'NORMAL' BOX

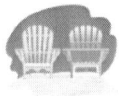

It sometimes felt like my whole childhood was dedicated to playing sports; constantly going to practices and games. As I got older it had consisted of up to one to two hours, three to five days a week. When my father was on the road, it was my mother's responsibility to take me to arena after arena, packing up my little sister, trusting that she was cozy and warm as she tagged along with us inside the cold ice rinks and sometimes unbearable blizzard travel nights. It never occurred to me just how much stress my schedule had added to my mother's already overloaded responsibilities.

But once my father arrived back home, weekdays and weekends were reserved for either running to hockey practices or assisting with coaching my games.

My family attended my hockey tournaments, as everyone else's families on my hockey team had; everyone looked forward to these experiences, bonding with teammates, their siblings, and their families. But as the years went by, my teammates' siblings grew older and were no longer as little as they once were. It began feeling harder to comprehend that although my sister was growing up alongside them - as they were the same age, she was still a little kid compared to the other siblings.

After our games, during our bonding activities (these were the moments, I'm pretty sure we had gotten into more trouble by the hotel staff than our own parents), I began noticing that the siblings were now old enough to hangout more independently from their parents. Whether they were bundled up in someone's hotel room watching movies and eating heaps of junk food, swimming in the hotel pool, or even playing ball hockey in the nearby hallway, they never considered inviting my sister. Looking back, I'm not sure how much they even interacted with her. Instead, my sister was in our hotel room watching a movie with my parents by herself, without any of my other teammate's siblings.

She wasn't included or invited in any of the activities with the other children.

To this day, it still saddens me that I had to witness my sister sit alone, excluded by the other children. It's like it happens over and over again, people think it's difficult to communicate or interact with my sister because she can't get out her words or move without a special aid. Judgment sets in, and they don't even try with her.

I realized I could have been more helpful to include her in things that she was capable of doing with us. I'm sure if I would have brought attention to how my sister was being excluded, I knew some of my teammates would have tried to do their best to include her.

Reflecting on these moments, I think I didn't say anything because of my own insecurities and maybe I was afraid that if I did mention it, they could have said no, or worse, they could've completely ignored me and turned around walking away, annoyed that I even asked.

"*If your happiness depends on the actions of others, you're at mercy of things that you can't control.*"

-Kendall Jenner

LESSONS FROM THE SHADOW

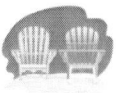

If I could offer one piece of advice, it would be to never take this special life we were born into for granted. It has taught me so many life lessons that have shaped me into the person that I am today. I question myself often where I would've ended up if I wasn't gifted this life with my sister.

This life has gifted me wisdom and expanded my heart. For many years, I used to resent this life, I used to think, *"Why me? Why does my family have to go through this? Why should my sister have to suffer? How would my parents take care of their child as if she were a toddler her whole life, let alone the difficulties it will be when she matures into adulthood."* I thought as we grew older it would become more difficult for me to explain that although she doesn't look like a child anymore, she still thinks and acts like one.

I believe that special needs children are born into our lives for a reason. They choose us, whether it was for them to teach us important life lessons or because God knew we would do anything in our power to give them a fulfilled life. We'd be their protector, love them, and accept them better than anyone else. Maybe our lesson is about how to love, whether that's for others or the love that we need to give to ourselves. They teach us how to slow down, to be in the present moment because life is too short to be stuck in the past or too far into the future. They teach us how to observe a person with kindness. They teach you to think about others more than you think about yourself, and when you become more sensitive, you begin to fully understand the whole in-depth meaning behind "put yourself in their shoes."

Never judge someone just by how you think you perceive them. We are all different, unique in our own way, trying to figure out this thing we all call life. If you haven't yet learnt this by now, I just hope you one day realize how privileged we all are to be here on this earth: to just be alive. Associating with anyone who has a disability could be equally as impactful on your life, just as you could lift and impact theirs, too. These generous, loved filled souls, who, regardless of what you mean to them, will show you what God's love truly feels like; being accepted and appreciated every single day, even if it's hard for them to show you or for you to notice.

Over time, I had learned to never feel embarrassed about my family's situation because the truth is, if people really judged my sister, thinking she was peculiar, then maybe we were better without them in our lives.

I've had to endure my own grief of not having the same life as my peers. I've always had a tight knit relationship with both my parents where I could be transparent and open about my thoughts, ideas, and emotions. But once my sister was born, it seemed to be a challenge for me to be open and honest with them about what I was going through. Some conversations became more difficult to communicate how I had felt during particular periods in my life, inducing many arguments I had with both my mother and father.

I'd bring up a situation, or rather I was complaining about something I had disagreed with, and my parents would often look at me and say, "Kylee, consider what it would feel like for them," not agreeing at all with what I had to say. They brought me back into this reality every time. I grew up into the mindset of 'stop just thinking about yourself' - even as a young child.

Every time I had this conversation with them, the more enraged I'd become, and the more I would lash out because I was annoyed that they wouldn't listen to my point of view. I felt like I was always in the wrong and I should put my feet in their shoes and get over it. I felt so hurt and betrayed. Eventually, I kept everything in because I felt like my parents had enough on their plate.

I had felt like I wasn't being heard and that I needed to always think of how the other person felt even if my feelings weren't being validated, like my feelings didn't amount to what the other person may have felt. I forced myself to believe that even if I didn't do anything to the person to feel a certain way, I knew that I needed to understand what the other person was feeling or going through in their life during this particular time.

They were trying to teach me empathy, but neglected to allow my feelings, needs and opinions to matter as much as everyone else's.

In truth, I was being heard; my parents just wanted me to be the bigger person, to be the kinder person. One of the lessons I had taken from this was, even though I have a complicated life, and it can be a very emotional roller coaster, unfortunately there's always someone experiencing something worse. It teaches you to appreciate everything, even finding the light in the darkness.

Honestly, I wouldn't trade this life for anything. I realized that fighting with the closest people in my life only made matters worse, especially when they were already going through their own daily stresses themselves. One of my biggest regrets was not being there for my family in the way I was supposed to. Even if I simply offered more of a helping hand or noticed and appreciated them for giving me their generous time and energy, when all they really needed was a break to recoup. Maybe, they just needed a hug, someone to tell them that they are appreciated and that I understand they're doing the best they can. Yet, my parents made sure to keep me and my sister active and they were heavily involved in our everyday life. For this, I thank them endlessly because sometimes it was the only thing that made me happy during the stressful times.

Throughout my life, almost all of my parents' attention was on my sister and all of her needs. It felt lonely at times, and I wished people would have checked up on me.

I was never ignored, my mother always asked me how I was. She asked me to open up, giving me permission to speak what was really on my mind, but the problem was no one had the solutions. My parents expressed they felt the same way.

It was not like anyone could turn around and change our life, our world was different and there was nothing we could do to change that.

But I wish they had held space for me to be honest, to feel heard without the tendency to always think of others. Sometimes you want to know that even if things can't change, it's okay to wish life were easier without feeling guilty for expressing it within the moments of grief.

And I wish the rest of the world, once in a while, asked about me; thought about me. It often felt like my feelings weren't valid because I don't have the same struggles as my sister. People didn't think to ask me, "How are you?" They worry about my sister, they sometimes think about my parents, but very few people think of the sibling. After all, our life isn't hard. But I still am affected by the struggles our family has to deal with. I feel all the pain, their worry, and it becomes my own.

I have to navigate both worlds - special needs, and the rest of the world separately; and yet it feels like I'm completely alone on both sides. Not able to fully relate to my peers, and on the side of special needs, always feeling the impact of the barriers placed on us; always being restricted because of my sibling's difficulties.

I was always asked to put my frustration aside because we were doing the best we could to navigate both worlds as a family. After all, there was nothing we could do to change our circumstance.

I had to just figure out how to set aside my desires, my wants, in the space of special needs. In the world the rest of society lives in, I was the one watching on the side lines as everyone blissfully lived their 'normal' lives not realizing how easy they had it; the simple things in life were my family's struggles and no one could change that, or maybe no one cared to see.

With time, I also discovered that assuming that people are judging you based on the fact that your family is different from others, is totally false! You and your family are unique in each and every way and that's okay- brilliant even! If people can't see that, then they are not worth being in your life.

Never stop being you. Be there for your family when they need you, trust your intuition, and never be afraid to meet new people and tell them about your own story- how you are honoured to be the sibling to this incredible human who happens to be differently abled. Be proud of it and who you've become along the way. I implore you to look for the opportunities where there is the freedom to ask questions, and then ask them! Don't be afraid to speak out, have strong opinions, let people hear your voice because it is powerful when used in the right way.

"You can't change someone who doesn't see an issue in his actions."

-OurMindLife.com

STOP ASKING WHAT'S WRONG WITH HER!

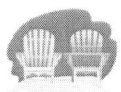

One of the hardest things a child could go through is growing up without a father around. My father's job required that he traveled far away from home, sometimes months at a time, leaving my mother to take care of me and my sister alone. This was especially difficult for our family.

I depended highly on my father to be the person that lifted my spirits and put a smile on my face. We'd laugh the kind of laugh that's deep in the pit of your stomach, making your eyes water with tears, when I needed it the most. He was the person who'd get me out of the house when the moments were too hard, and I needed a distraction. Most importantly, I needed him at times to be there for me when my mother couldn't because her attention was given to my sister. But the truth was my sister needed her attention more than I ever did; twenty-four-seven in order to survive because she couldn't do things on her own.

My mother fed her, brushed her teeth, bathed her, dressed her, washed her hands, and scheduled her toileting. My mother always kept her occupied and protected at all times-she never took her eyes off of her. It was hard enough to get a babysitter or a nanny because we had difficulties trusting anyone to care for her complex needs, and it would be difficult for her to communicate to us if something had happened with these people since she is nonverbal. To this day, my sister still and will always until she is old and grey, depend highly on my mother not only for her self-care, but to be her advocate, her eyes, her ears, and her voice.

As I grew older and reflected back on moments throughout my childhood, I remembered all the times I had taken my mother's efforts for granted, when she was there to cook, clean, keep us safe, make us feel loved always, and continually made sure we got to experience the things both my sister and I were interested in, even if it wasn't easy all the time.

My parents dedicated their time, patience, dollars, and life into my sports interests, school events, hosted my birthday parties, and made sure that I had fun and memorable adventures with my friends. But even with all of their efforts to give me a "normal life", I still lost who I was. I lost how to be a good sister and even a caring daughter. I had become embarrassed by the person I was turning into. I thought if people saw that my family was different, they were going to not like me, or they'd judge me and leave- I was terrified I would be the lonely kid that no one would want to be associated with. For some reason I had this fear that they'd be ashamed to be around me knowing I was from that family with the special needs kid. It's difficult for me to admit this, but I began looking at my family as a disappointment and an embarrassment rather than a blessing.

I had a lot of childhood friends growing up who were all very sheltered like I was. They were very kind-hearted, genuine, and spoke nicely to my sister. These were my friends before my sister was born. I never had to answer their endless questions and stares when they were newly in the presence of my sister. They already knew the answers because they were part of my sister's journey of discovering her truths, watching her struggles, listening to our concerns and fears that we had for her. They held her on their laps, hugged her, and spoke loving words to her when she was a baby and continued that loving respect even as my sister's complex needs began uncovering themselves to the world. These friends took my whole family in, and they accepted and cared for us without judgment. When it came to our up and down moments, they knew when we needed that extra support and encouragement to stay strong and to be hopeful.

However, as I got older and my social circle expanded and once I started to introduce these new peers into my life, questions from them followed about my sister. Eventually it started to become harder and harder bringing new people into our home and into my family's life knowing I had to answer questions that clearly outed my sister's disability. It was difficult for me confronting the fact that they, already within minutes of meeting her, recognized something was different and that she had a disability because of her actions. The minute we walked out of the room that my sister was in, they would drill me with questions that I didn't want to answer, I didn't want to explain it to someone who I was just getting to know.

"I don't want this to sound rude but what's wrong with your sister. What does she have?" Or even plainly, "What's wrong with her?" It was awful- *what's wrong with her!*

What's wrong with you!? Let's ask deep questions about your life, about your family!

Of course I didn't say that, and I knew our lives weren't ever going to be the same. Instead, I held my head down, as my heart sank with so much sadness for my sister. Parts of me started breaking into pieces every time I would hear those words, and I thought about how I should explain how awesome she is to them and that she isn't her disability.

Would they see her in all her beauty rather than just seeing her with all her needs?

Every time this happened, it was like another thick and heavy layer of sadness floated around me for my sister- knowing that to other people she was always going to have a label.

A part of me was concerned that after I answered my new friends' questions, would they act weirdly towards my sister and me now? Were they watching us, paying close attention to us, to decipher if there were any similarities or differences between us. Would they look at me and wonder the same, if it's something we both have? Is it in my DNA? Was there something wrong with me, was there something wrong with my parents too?

Like, what did they think she had? A contagious disease? Why was it so common for this question to be asked this way? Can't you just see her without a disability! Whether it is out of genuine curiosity, sometimes it didn't feel that way. It almost felt like some sort of attack on the truth about our family and our life.

I began to accept that everyone, including myself at times, has a deep desire to uncover the answers to everything - it's a known fact. It doesn't matter what it is, we are searching for the label. We want to place things in order, so we feel better about how we are understanding our environments. We want to have meaning for what we can't make sense of.

When you live in our world and have to experience these kinds of conversations so many times, with so many different people, it becomes frustrating. It's extremely upsetting constantly needing to explain. It's like my sister is the elephant in the room and everyone is asking, why is this person different? Everyone is asking what is wrong with her- why can't people allow her disability to be a normal thing?

When talking to families about their situation, often it can be a hard topic for them to discuss. Not everyone understands what it's like to take care of someone for the rest of your life. Not everyone understands what it's like to be in our shoes, or to be my sister and to feel what she goes through everyday of her life. Imagine doctors, strangers, colleagues, neighbours, community members, family members, friends, therapists, teachers, strangers, or the kids at the park, all noticing and openly asking and relying on you to explain why she's different, and often right in front of my sister! You begin to feel annoyed and tired of answering people's pretentious demands for answers. You want to scream at them, *"You are an asshole!"* She understands. Imagine if people continually asked what's wrong with you just because you are being you!

It was too much for all of us to handle and I can't imagine how my sister felt! I was uncomfortable with what defined "special needs", and the truth was, I was still learning what it really meant. What it meant to me - not the world's definition of special needs, because it was obvious they were misunderstanding it.

"Why fit in when you were born to stand out?"

-Dr. Seuss

STOP STARING, IT'S RUDE

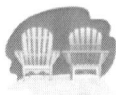

Why do people stare is a question I've repeatedly asked myself. Are we staring out of curiosity, jealousy, annoyance, disgust or judgment? Sometimes you might not even be aware you're doing it; a natural habit that we humans do on a daily basis.

For me, staring had a whole different meaning. Once my sister was born, it no longer felt innocent, the stares felt more like disgust and disapproval. I feel like my family has lived through enough stares to last a lifetime.

A simple trip to the grocery store; one of us pushing my sister in her wheelchair while the other was in charge of the grocery cart, and of course as I observed my surroundings, there was always someone who had stopped what they were doing to stare at us. I remember angrily screaming at them in my head, *"like, do you know that she's well aware that you're looking at her, judging her? She has feelings, too, you know!"*

I remember countless times we'd be enjoying ourselves in a restaurant and my sister would shout out a loud noise, and I swear the entire restaurant stopped what they were doing and looked over at our table - almost irritated that we disrupted their dinners with my sister's unintentional outburst. I remember feeling so embarrassed as the whole restaurant was staring at us; their glares felt like they were mentally saying "how dare we bring her into the restaurant and let her screech like that!"

These outbursts were the one thing about my sister I had struggled with the most growing up. I really didn't understand it, and I didn't know how to block everyone's negative reactions towards it.

Some people found it difficult to understand that not all that we may consider inappropriate behaviour, is a result of out-of-control children or lazy parenting.

For some individuals, like my sister, their brain has difficulty sometimes making sense of their environment; the different stimuli their brain is trying to process and make sense of - everything we don't know we are even doing every second of the day. Things like making sense of different temperatures we touch or foods we put in our mouth, the different surfaces we touch, hearing unexpected loud noises, and even visual input - the information our brain is receiving from our eyes; our nervous system perceives and processes all these stimuli at once. Through the experiential learning process, a healthy brain understands what it needs to do with the information coming in. However, for the person who has a sensory processing difficulty, these simple and usually quite pleasurable experiences, can feel overwhelming and can cause a lot of distress for the individual.

When my sister was younger, it was sometimes difficult for her brain to manage and understand the sensory input she was experiencing, sometimes inducing feelings of overwhelm for her. This internal chaos displayed itself as short explosive reactions, which of course were judged by others, assuming she was a child acting out. Today, it seems as though her brain has learned to perceive and process much easier, and many of the explosive responses she struggled with no longer surface as often.

However, she does continue to have moments when, out of the blue, and with no warning or understandable reason, she shouts a short and loud *"aaaa"* sound, and afterwards she appears upset and disappointed in herself that it just happened. Both my parents and I believe that it seems like it's a compulsive action, perhaps like that of someone with Tourette's; but unlike someone who unintentionally shouts a word, she shouts a sound because she is nonverbal.

Sometimes, in rare occasions when my sister is extremely excited, she demonstrates a peculiar reaction. In these moments, she tucks her arms bent and tight to the sides of her chest while her hands open and close rapidly, her breathing shallow - almost as if she is hyperventilating, and because her mouth is open and shaped like an O, an *"ough"* sounds explodes out of her. For a very long time I struggled with these reactions. I was embarrassed, even though we all knew that this was an action done through compulsion and she had difficulty stopping. I even remember my parents saying that one of my sister's therapists witnessed one of these episodes, and she even asked, *"What was that?"* Not understanding Mikaela's episode either, she, in fact, commented that she wondered if her brain was in a looped response in that moment.

Over time, I began realizing that the staring was just people observing out of wonder, and my anxiety surrounding my sister's behaviour subsided as I gained the understanding around what my sister was experiencing. Each reaction was actually informing us on how she was feeling; fear, frustration, pain, overly excited; they all appeared differently.

It's my opinion that people need to be more consciously aware when they stare. Learn to be kinder; smile, say hello, speak to the person with the disability and to their family. Don't look away like you're embarrassed because when you do this, that actually makes us feel worse. It makes us feel like you think there is something so wrong with us that you refuse to acknowledge our presence. Would you stare at other families like you stare at mine? Would you stare and look away without even a smile? A simple smile, and perhaps a hello, goes a long way in helping people feel like they matter. Remember that there may be more going on beneath the surface that both the child and family may be coping with. Please be compassionate and observe with kind eyes.

Not only do you affect how the family feels when you refuse to acknowledge them, but I've seen how this also affects my sister. I've witnessed her transform into an introverted shy kid, afraid of being noticed and being judged. We've even experienced several incidents when a person attempted to say hello and make conversation with my sister instead of looking away, but once they realized she doesn't speak, they usually seem uncomfortable and don't know what to do or say next, so they say nothing at all and walk away. Imagine how this would feel; you are trying to communicate with another person, and they look at you strangely and walk away from you, without a response, explanation or a goodbye. There are so many moments I can recall catching myself witnessing someone staring at my little sister, and my initial instincts were to glare back at them.

I can remember my little nine-year-old self standing there, leaning forward on my tip toes as I stared at them; looking into their soul with rage, my face hardened, my eyes squinted, my brows furrowed, and my teeth clenched together. But they didn't even notice me! They were just looking at her, and at the time, I interpreted these stares as judgment; it infuriated me! I truly believed in those moments I was going to teach them a lesson, but instead, it didn't. It only taught me one.

"Everybody is a genius.
But if you judge a fish by its
ability to climb a tree,
it will live its whole life
believing that
it is stupid."

-Albert Einstein

DID THAT JUST REALLY HAPPEN?

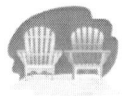

Lady, You Are Pathetic

It was the beginning of October, and the sights of fall were everywhere and so was the Halloween decor in the stores. My sister was eager to go to the Halloween store to purchase a new costume for the upcoming trick or treating night. Our family walked into the store, adoring my sister beaming with excitement. As we strolled through each aisle, my sister was intent on saying hello as each child intermingled around us, all just as enthused about the Halloween inspired atmosphere as my sister was.

It seemed as if the children weren't as receptive to my sister's friendliness, and to her dismay, they weren't quick to reciprocate her kind gestures. As she gently reached out her hand to say hello to a little kid, the mother, with a petrified look on her face, shoved her (what appeared to be her four-year-old) away from my sister's reach, purposely blocking my sister from being able to touch her children! It was like the women didn't understand or see my sister's kindness. To our family it had felt like she shoved her children away as if my sister had some sort of 'contagious disease' and she was convinced they would absorb it from her touch. The mother quickly moved them into another aisle so my sister wasn't around them. My sister was trying to say, "Hi guys! Isn't this place awesome, look at all these cool things!"

Instead, my mother had to reassure my sister, "Don't worry hunny, that lady was weird", trying to distract her from the woman's odd and inappropriate behaviour.

It seems that even today, parents are still not acknowledging the importance of teaching their children that everyone should be treated with kindness. All people, not just the people who look and act the same as you. Whether the person has a disability or not, treat people with dignity, respect, and kindness.

Everyone has feelings, everyone wants to be valued and appreciated. No one should ever feel discriminated against just because they have a disability. Parents who choose to avoid having these conversations with their children about people who have special needs, are only teaching their vulnerable children to view this community through misunderstood perceptions.

It could be possible that it's coming from a place of fear that is held within yourself from generational programming from your own parents and society. Maybe disability is something you've never quite understood, something that you are not sure how to explain because no one has had this conversation with you.

By avoiding these conversations with your children, you make your own children feel uncomfortable and afraid to be around people who are differently abled. You are not dissolving generational false and detrimental beliefs that have been wrongfully attached to the special needs community.

Instead, you are ensuring continued exclusion, discrimination, and pain for these individuals and for their families.

I Relate to You

It had only been the third time in over six years that I had watched a hockey game. As I sat in the stands, I observed my surroundings, and I began noticing many children and young adults with special needs at the game cheering and supporting our hometown's junior hockey team. A few kids were even past teammates from my sister's baseball league.

The head coach for the home team was my sister's public-school teacher. And I pondered if the kids that were in the stands around me were either present students or even previous students of his.

On my right and a few bleacher sections away, was a man in his mid-to-late twenties who from the looks of it, was the older brother accompanied by his special needs sibling. I observed how he interacted with his brother. I was worried from personal experience, that he would notice that I was looking at them. I knew what the stares felt like, and I was afraid that he would think I was judging them.

This young man reminded me a lot of my sister and it appeared that every time he was excited, he would get louder and louder.

At this moment, I was curious about how the older brother was handling the strangers' reactions towards his brother's behaviours.

At certain moments, I could almost feel him as if he was thinking, "No, not right now, please stop staring". He began looking down, and sometimes he'd stare straight at the ice trying to ignore and normalize his brother's loud yelling and trying to erase the stares from the strangers looking at them.

I wondered if the older brother felt like I had so many times before, wishing he didn't have the thoughts of, "Why now? Not here. I love you, but please don't make loud noises here."

It shouldn't have mattered how loud he was. We were in an arena; everyone was loud.

People need to start asking themselves, would I like it if someone stared at me the way I am staring?

I wished I would have sat closer to them so I could have smiled at them and said hello to them both. I would have made a light conversation, and I would have done my best to let them know, "Yes, I see you're happy and it's so awesome! I appreciate you and I get it."

Appalling Actions Towards My Sister Has Been Displayed by Even the Young

When I was a teenager, I witnessed yet another incident involving my sister and a younger boy. It was the first situation where I really had no clue how to handle the child's unexpected behaviour. We stopped in to quickly say hello to my mother's old neighbourhood friend. Her son was home from daycare and already at play in his playroom, so my sister and I joined in too. I had left the playroom for a few minutes and when I returned, the little boy was standing in front of my sister. He looked at me, smiled mischievously and said, "Hey, do you wanna see something funny? When I do this, she gets scared." Without physically hitting her, he thought it was hilarious to tease her like he was going to swing his plastic sword at her face just to watch her flinch in terror, and then he broke out in laughter.

My sister flinched out of fear, fear that he was going to hit her right in the face! She doesn't have quick reflexes and can't protect herself from getting bluntly hit by his sword. With no way of blocking her own face, she closed her eyes hoping he wouldn't actually hit her.

At the time I was too young, I didn't know how to handle this situation, but I definitely knew it wasn't okay! I remember taking the sword away from him and saying, "Don't do that!" After that, I didn't leave my sister's side as we waited for my mother to finish her visit. On the car ride home, I began telling my mother what had happened. That was the very last time we saw them.

The truth was in this scenario, it had felt harder to know how to handle the situation properly especially because I didn't know this family well, and because of the fact that he was only three years old! Looking back, I should have said, "No we don't do that, you don't hurt people." And I definitely should have taken my sister where my mother was so she was safe, I don't know why I didn't tell my mother earlier and while we were there, but I think it was because I was terrified to leave my sister alone and it was too hard for me to physically move her, so that we, together, could find my mother.

This experience shocked us all and we no longer trusted anyone.

Funny... I Think Not!

When I was at the age where I could drive alone with my peers, I commonly heard jokes about parking in the accessible parking spots. Even if they were the nicest person in the world, in most cases they were clueless about how their jokes would upset me or frustrate me even though it had just fallen out of their mouths; it made me look at them from a different perspective.

I wondered if it was safe to have them in my life and around my family. I worried how they would perceive my family. Would they judge my sister and make fun of her behind my back?

It never failed, we would pile into someone's vehicle and pull up into a Walmart parking lot and the person in the driver's seat would say, "Let's park in the handicap parking spot. Everyone get out of the car and act retarded so we can be closer to the door."

Regretfully in those moments, I stayed silent, shocked by the reality of what they thought was funny and unsure how I was supposed to express how morally wrong their jokes were. Holding onto the fear of being excluded if I voiced my truth. I was alone after all, in this world of disability and I was afraid that no one would respect or understand what I had to say.

Oops... Sorry I Shouldn't Have Said That

In the dictionary, the word retarded means less advanced in mental, physical, or social development than is usual for one's age. Why is this word still being used today? Why is it still so easy for people to throw around the word retard and joke about it?

For centuries, people with special needs have been stigmatized with names; moron, feeble-minded, retarded, stupid, idiot, dull, slow. In Wikipedia, intellectual disability (also defined as general learning disability or intellectual learning disability) is described as mental retardation.

How is it still described as this in the 21st century, when we are advocating strongly for all human rights? Voicing loudly the acknowledgment that we are all equal and people are declaring, "There will be an end to discrimination!" What about the community of special needs? Clearly there has not been enough acknowledgment in society to recognize the need to support this change!

Nothing is worse than overhearing conversations happening with people you know, and all of a sudden, that word falls out of their mouth. They catch themselves saying it, but it's too late. Then they look in your direction with a guilty face, because they realize who they said the word in front of. Their head drops low, and their gaze leaves your eyes as they admit they shouldn't use that word. They may be saying this in a way to apologize for possibly offending you, but all it does is makes it clear that they think your sibling with special needs is retarded!

The word retarded has caused so many layers of generational pain and years of discrimination. This community has experienced isolation, hatred, abandonment, abuse, alienation, and they have even been viewed as a burden on their families and society at large. The only way for society to truly heal this community is to abandon the word retarded entirely and to never use this word again!

It should never be used as a joke or to be used to describe someone who has an intellectual disability. I realize this is a lot to ask since this word has been a part of our culture and used to not just describe someone with an intellectual disability, but we use it to describe an individual who is acting as if they have an intellectual disability; someone who is not acting with their full intelligence.

We have all used it, including myself - never in a malicious way, but as slurs in a joke towards a friend who's making a spectacle of themselves. But in writing this book and really diving deep into my life, my sister's life, and realizing how much this word affects the special needs community, it's clear to me change needs to take place. I am choosing to no longer use this word; I am removing it from my vocabulary, and I implore you to do the same.

"Allow yourself to let go of the people, thoughts, and situations that poison your well-being. Love yourself enough to create an environment in your life that is conducive to the nourishment of your personal growth."

-Steve Maraboli

DATING WHEN YOU HAVE A SPECIAL NEEDS SIBLING

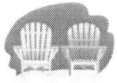

How is dating when you have a special seeds sibling, you may be wondering?

Well, dating can be complicated especially when keeping your special needs sibling in mind. Whether you are dating or not, when you bring someone into your life, they get to know your family on a personal level and may possibly one day have a relationship with. Someone who could become part of your family unit, so it's important that they blend well.

Whoever I choose to bring into my life, I have an expectation that they never judge me or my family. It's usual for me to have my guard up when I meet new people, in fear that they will become close to my family and then out of the blue they leave, never talking to us again.

I have a rule I made for myself and the people I bring into my family; until I know you are trustworthy and are close enough for me to share this part of my life with, I keep you out of my sister's life. I would find myself leaving out of the conversation that my sister has a disability until I was comfortable with trusting the person, and how they viewed the special needs community. I used to think of this as a protection mechanism for both my sister and for myself.

What I discovered later was that this shield I put up was not always the best way of starting a new friendship or even a new relationship. But I have learned through experience that not everyone that enters your life has the best intentions. They may not even care about getting to know your family, and so being mindful, and listening to your intuition is imperative.

One time, I was talking to this one guy, let's call him John. After having several conversations with him, John showed me a version of himself that I couldn't look past - a version of himself I wasn't expecting. At the beginning of us getting to know each other, the exchange brought laughter and fun banter. We were both eager to get to know each other a little more, and I wanted to see what kind of person he really was, so I asked him what type of humour he had.

Since I'd never really met him before, and we were only texting on our iPhones, I thought it was another way for me to test him; to get to know him better. I ask this because I've discovered that humour shows a lot about a person's character.

John answered back with, "I have kind of a weird sense of humour, it's slightly dark." At this point after reading this, I wasn't sure what I was walking into. His version of expressing his humour was through 'MEMES '- I had no idea what this meant. Within seconds, six pictures (MEMES) showed up on my phone screen, as I gazed over the jokes, I couldn't stop staring at the third MEME. A picture of a Caucasian young female with a darker young male whom both had

Down Syndrome, the words on the picture were "mixed vegetables". I thought to myself, this is what "John" really thought was funny? This was his humour?

This can't be real; people don't actually make fun of people with special needs, do they? I wondered. I was infuriated and lost in my own thoughts about what just took place. I ended up completely ignoring him because I couldn't collect my thoughts to articulate how wrong that was all while trying to calm my anger.

I had pondered over ideas for the next few days about how I would bring forth this difficult conversation with him. I felt the urge to tell him how much of an awful human being he was and to demand he never talk to me again.

I felt so uncomfortable to even say, *"Dude, you don't know this about me, but I have a special needs sibling, and I am extremely offended with what you just sent me!*

Why would you actually think this is funny? You're an ignorant and awful person!"

What was he going to say to that? "Okay?" Or "I am so sorry, I didn't know. I feel so bad". Or just DELETE, never hearing a response from him again.

As each day passed by with no explanation to my disappearance, I wondered what would have happened if I had just told him the truth about how I felt. Would it have made a significant difference in the way he viewed himself?

Would it have changed his perspective regarding differently abled persons? Maybe he would have an epiphany moment and notice how his actions have an effect on other people. The truth was, he had no idea that what he thought was funny, was actually extremely offensive and wrong. He also didn't know that I had a special needs sibling.

During my long attempt to ignore him, he still wouldn't leave me alone, asking what he did wrong or why I was ignoring him. So, I finally brought up the courage and told him the truth. It felt like a truck load of anxiety had just lifted off my shoulders. To say the least, I learned a lot from this experience, and I started to use this question as a way of gauging a person, testing them before I get to close to them.

I met this other guy on a date and funnily enough, I had asked him the same question, what is your sense of humour?

He told me that his mother was a therapist who works with people with special needs, "My mother likes to call me her, "special boy", because she says that the way I act and joke around, reminds her of her clients. But she never likes using the word reta**d because it would be rude against her clients", he noted. He sent me random videos that he took of himself dancing and acting with lots of excessive energy, making a spectacle of himself.

Once again, I found myself bewildered by people's ignorance. What his mother said was very inappropriate and unprofessional, something no one, especially someone who works in that field should ever make fun of! All this video showed me was how weird this guy was. So obviously, yeah, pass, he's out!

I worried about things like what if my significant other is never able to understand what my sister is trying to say to him. What if I liked him so much but he turned out to be someone who had a really difficult time relating to her? And what if he wasn't interested in putting in the effort to want to learn, so he ignores her? The reality was, that if someone was like that, the relationship would have never worked. And so, I tested people early and if they didn't pass the test, they were out. It had to be this way for me and for my family.

In the past, I've had people in my life that would ignore my sister just because they were uncomfortable. I never wanted this to happen with the person I wanted to be with, and I prayed I wouldn't have to teach 'the person I was meant to be with' how to communicate with my sister. I hoped it would just come naturally for them. I chose to trust that the right person would just get it. It would be simple and their interaction with my sister would be as natural as breathing for them.

It turns out that with time, I found that this person does exist.

"I feel like a part of my soul has loved you since the beginning of everything. Maybe we're from the same star."

- Emery Allen

MY BABY SISTER

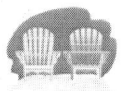

Oh, my sweet baby sister, how you've grown up, the beautiful young women that you have become. I wish I could go back and slow down life, reliving the best moments of our childhood together again. Watching you grow up through the lens from which I view my life today.

As a child, my relationship with my sister wasn't always the simplest, nor am I proud of how I acted as her sibling.

Throughout the process of writing this book, revealing memories I've tried to tuck away and forget, it made me realize how many moments that I wish I could have taken back and do over. I've held so much guilt for looking at her like she was different, and because of her, I wasn't going to live what I considered a normal life.

During my childhood, I had resented my sister. I blamed her for my family's sadness, all the times I heard the word 'no' from my parents, and for making our family so different from everyone else's. I misunderstood her and I knew that because society pressured me to seek an independent life from her, I didn't understand how I fit within the world of special needs. It was confusing to me.

People constantly asked, "What is she diagnosed with? "

And as a kid, I noticed how everyone was so apprehensive to ask the question, but you could sense their desperate curiosity to know the answer. I could see the tension they held in their body and in their face as they asked about my sister. I could feel their worry for her and for my parents. At the same time, I could tell these interactions for my mother brought up feelings of grief. I could tell she was so desperately trying to hide. It was terrifying and confusing to witness as a kid, and it made me feel so unstable. Then, to add to the pain of that uncomfortable question, they would respond by saying, "Oh, I am so sorry."

Really! Why scare me even more? Thanks.

In time, what I discovered was that what truly matters most in my life is my family. Without my sister, life would be unfathomable. I can't picture my life any other way and I don't want to.

Once we had moved and started traveling with my father, our relationship as a family changed as a whole. I always wondered, had it not been for our travels, being stuck in hotel rooms together, would we be close with each other the way we are now? We may appear different on the outside, but our personalities are so similar. Had we not acquired this tight knit bond that we have today, would we not know how much we were in need of each other's company? Would we have been close at all?

As we traveled, I began observing my sister, realizing that there were a lot of similarities in her that I saw in myself. I influenced her even when at the time I didn't think she understood me. I'd joke with her, and she would laugh at the appropriate times. There was so much more to my sister than I had noticed before - she was hilarious! I began appreciating how lucky I was to have her as my sibling.

Watching her as she communicates to other people with disabilities, and how she just knows what they need to feel seen was an amazing lesson for me to experience. She uses her physical touch; a gentle open hand on the shoulder or cheek, as she leans slightly forward making eye contact with them, almost as if she's connecting to their inner thoughts. When she does this to me, I feel the intention and the love that she emits from her thoughts.

She is my example of how to live life through the lens of empathy. It makes me melt with gratitude and I am so in awe of how she always just knows who needs this type of physical interaction; it's her way of communicating to them, and their response is magical. She's letting them know that she sees them, she is connecting with them. That she understands them and that they are being heard. It's her way of acknowledging them, loving them, and for her to show them that she cares. She even does this with me whenever she sees me cry in front of her, it's an instant calming connection. I know my sister will never judge me, but instead love me for who I am, not just because I am her sister, but because of who she is as a person.

"Be yourself. Everyone else is taken."

-Oscar Wilde

DEAR BABY SISTER

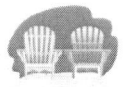

Dear baby sister, you loving, sweet, caring being. As I sat there on the hospital bed beside our mother after you were born, holding you in my arms, I knew you came into my life to change the way I would see this world - in a whole new light, with a whole new perspective.

I love that you try to copy me and like to experience the things that I am interested in. You make me so proud to be your big sister.

We may at times both have separation anxiety every time we're away from one another, but then argue when we are together like a typical 'normal' sister relationship. I like getting to know all the different versions of you that makes you, you. I will always take your angry days, upset days, and your happy ones too.

I want you to never feel like you have to be someone else when you're around others, because once you're around people, the truth is, they can't help but adore you. I love you and I am forever grateful to be your big sister.

I witnessed you become the class clown and Miss Popular in every grade you graduated from. You were loved for your unconditional kindness and your endless ability to get along and include everyone, and you lit up every room with your presence. Baby sister, you have the kindest soul, and somehow you make everyone in our life feel better without saying a word.

Wondering "*What If*", Doesn't Make You a Bad SIB

Sometimes I can't help but wonder what my sister would have been like if she had no disability at all. What would be on her mind, would she have a million things to say? Would her voice be different when she talked in clear sentences?

What would she do with her life if she had the freedom to live on her own? I always dreamed of us having girls' night, doing facials or painting our nails as we binged watched our new favourite Netflix series while laughing about the boys we liked. And I've daydreamed what it would feel like as a big sister helping her get ready for her first date or her prom. Would she let me help her with her makeup and hair? Would it have been like the movies where we build these special little memories together bonding over these adolescent milestones?

"Just because someone carries it well doesn't mean it isn't heavy."

-Unknown

FINALLY GETTING MY MOTHER BACK

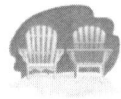

Once we had moved, traveling became something I had looked forward to. My mother had enough of being apart from my father for so long, and raising my sister and me frequently on her own had put a toll on our entire family.

Within a blink, it felt like years were flying by and my father was missing our childhood. When the idea of moving turned into an option, they had both felt like it would be the best opportunity to support our family. Wherever my father would go we would be there with him, job to job, state to state. It was as if my family was 're-united' for what felt like the first time in a long time. Life was finally starting to feel normal.

My father's constant travels never stopped, there were some years where he was away for several weeks, even months at a time without seeing him. He would come home for a weekend and have to leave again for a couple more months.

I never truly knew what it was like to have parents who worked a nine to five job and then came home at the end of each day - everyone gathering around the kitchen table to have a nice home cooked meal as a family.

When my father was home and we all had dinner together, it was as if it was a special occasion, something that we had all looked forward to.

I could tell my mother tried to wear her mask, hiding her depression from the world and from us. Pretending that she was okay when all she wanted was for my father to come home so she didn't feel so alone and overwhelmed. I never thought about how my father had felt, of course he wanted to be home, to be with us. But traveling was a part of his job and that was his way of taking care of us.

During the first couple years of traveling, I saw for the first time changes within my mother; she was beginning to beam with life again. If I am being honest, for a few years I thought I had lost her.

"In order to love who you are you cannot hate the experiences that shaped you. "

-Homebody Club

SHE'S NOT JUST MY FRIEND, SHE'S MORE LIKE MY SISTER

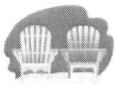

When I look at other sibling relationships, I can't help but envy them.

Although, I have a beautiful relationship with my sister and I would never trade what we have, at times it is so difficult to digest how different our relationship is compared to other siblings. This was especially difficult when we moved, and I lost all my friendships.

My life is different, and I accept all its challenges, but during moments of being alone, I contemplated if my sister ever feels the way I do. Did she depend on me to be her friend too?

Growing up I had this friend - I can't pinpoint exactly what made her different from the others, but out of all the fish in the sea, I would have chosen her to be my friend in every lifetime. She understood my life and knew how to connect with my sister when a lot of people didn't. Through all the highs and lows, she was always there for me- she was my other half; a second sister that I didn't realize how much I needed.

When I moved, we grew apart and I started to grieve her and her daily presence in my life, unable to figure out how I was going to live this life without her being a part of our family anymore.

How did my sister deal with her absence, too? I wondered if she noticed, if she questioned as to why she had left. Did she feel abandoned by her?

I wondered if her own parents noticed we weren't friends anymore, or if they really knew how important it was that we stay friends? Did they know that our friendship was truly valuable for me or how much of an impact she had on my life? She was more than a friend, she was like a sister. I wished they knew how her friendship filled a missing void that hasn't been replaced since we parted.

I wish my parents did more to keep that connection alive for us, but I think that early on they were dealing with so much that they didn't notice what was happening to our friendship. And when they did finally notice, it felt like too much time had passed and she was now living a full life without me.

I really wish that parents understood that when you're the only sibling to the child with special needs, it can be very lonely and isolating. If the sibling does find this kind of friendship that fills their missing void; the kind of kinship that should last forever, they need to take notice and do everything they can to support and foster your child's friendships. The SIB needs that support system. They need that person to rely on, to cry with, and someone to confide in - that person to be there for them no matter what.

Losing this friendship has been my biggest regret and continues to be one of my greatest voids in my life.

"If you are lucky enough to have a friend that has a sibling with special needs, hold onto her really tight and don't let her go!
She will be your best friend, biggest supporter, most trusted and real friend for life.
She will respect, accept, trust, and never judge you, believe in you, and always love you.
Friendship to her means unconditional love, support, fun, respect, and laughter.
She values every little smile, embrace, laugh, gesture, accomplishment, word, and so much more because she values and appreciates the details. These little gems fill her soul and creates a deeper love that is

unsurpassed! Be that for her too. And then, you will be the luckiest person on earth!"
-UNKNOWN

YOU CAN TRY TO RUN BUT YOU CAN'T HIDE

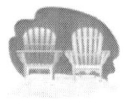

I, still to this day, find talking about my mental health very challenging. I often avoided facing the reality that I was suffering, especially from something I struggled to understand.

Since I was twelve, I have suffered from OCD (obsessive-compulsive disorder), depression, and anxiety. I tried so desperately to run and hide from facing the thoughts that were in my head; my inner demons that always made me believe that I was different and there was something wrong with me.

I didn't understand what was wrong with me, what was going on in my head, and why I felt so stuck thinking this way. I continually questioned myself, *"Why, why is this happening to me, why do I feel this way?"* I never could make sense of it, or reason with what was triggering the panic attacks and my on-going OCD episodes. At times, I felt trapped in an abyss of sadness and fear, and I concealed it behind my mask of smiles.

Once my sister was born, life looked a little different, and at a very young age I began acknowledging the expectations and pressures of what my future responsibilities as the sibling would likely require of me as I grew older. Without anyone pointing it out, I understood that one day I might be taking care of my elderly parents and also my elderly special needs sibling.

Maybe other siblings within the community of special needs have stared at this truth too, eyes wide open and thought *OMG* about this idea. It's understandable that the sibling's mental health might be challenged throughout the process of walking this path we have been given.

After researching about the siblings of a special needs child, I contemplated how much we conceal beneath the surface, hidden from all of those around us. Other siblings expressed the same fears I have had of bearing a child with special needs, especially after witnessing it with your own parents.

But the truth is, no one has answers. Just because you have a special needs sibling doesn't mean you will bear a child with special needs. In some cases, families who have no genetic mutations or family history of special needs, sometimes still end up carrying a child with a disability; anything could happen to the infant while developing, at birth, and sometimes years after. I would have appreciated knowing this and I wished that someone would have told me this when I was younger.

I battled between my fears and the part of myself that tried reassuring me that future was going to turn out the way I longed for. I thought that I needed to complete my OCD habits of tapping or touching something four or six times so I could feel satisfied enough to believe that nothing bad was going to happen. I worried about the people that were the closest to me, this was what caused me to have panic attacks. I feared if I didn't follow through with these compulsive urges that OCD consumes you with, something bad would happen. I was worried that I would be alone if I didn't do it.

Even though I knew logically this wasn't and never would be true, my brain looped and highjacked my capacity to stop doing it. My brain was compulsive, it was literally holding power over me, demanding that I follow through with these rituals in order to release the anxiety that was overwhelming me in the first place.

In all honesty, mental health can be difficult to understand. It may come from something deep within us, whether it is from past traumas or stresses that we continue to carry throughout our lifetime. You feel so alone, desperate to reach out but scared to even try. You may feel like you're going crazy, and no one will understand you; scared that your actions will make them run away because of how weird it seems. I had never felt so alone during this period of my life and my parents didn't know how to calm my fears. I was scared for the worst; a reality that was not even real.

In society, today it's very common for people to struggle with their mental health. Remember we are not alone; there is a likelihood that people around us struggle with their own inner demons; fighting their silent battles, believing the absolute worst, even if they're brilliant actors and you can't tell on their faces. The World Health Organization - Mental Disorders article states that, "One in every eight people in the world suffer with their mental health on a daily basis".

I figured out how to master the technique of disguising my OCD once I was around others who weren't my immediate family.

I continued to hide my emotions, keeping my thoughts, and feelings tucked away from the world.

I even feared speaking out to a professional because I thought, why would I go talk to them when they would never understand my life. What more do they know that I don't already know?

Even if I did reach out to people, it never felt like they really had the answers I needed; the words that made me feel better or the answers to my endless questions of "why". I started to believe no one could really relate to me, and there was nothing that a professional could contribute that would have pulled me out of my loneliness and changed our situation for our family.

I am not promoting that I made the correct choice. If anything, it couldn't be clearer to me today now after so many years struggling, that our whole family needed support from a professional. It would have likely helped us understand our grief and supported us through all the new surprises and unknowns that this life brings.

Please learn from my mistakes and seek help from a professional.

I know it isn't fair for me to say this or assume that a professional wouldn't have helped me, but if I really dive deep and question myself and my choice as to why I refused this kind of help, I knew it was because I didn't really want to face how I truly felt, I was ashamed, scared and I was secretly terrified of what they might say about me. I was too embarrassed to even receive the help.

So instead of accepting help, I found myself continuously getting lost in my thoughts and fears until I eventually exploded, and everyone saw the truth of how I really was behind the shadow of my sister. Only they were angry and looked at me like I was a spoiled brat who was selfishly seeking out for attention. "What more do I need that I don 't already have?" I'm guessing they wondered.

When you have a differently abled sibling, it's feasible to assume you have struggled with moments of feeling alone; maybe your sibling requires a lot of your parents' attention. Maybe you feel like no one is there to support you, that no one is there to console you, or hear you when you need to get something off your chest. You may feel like there's no one there for you to express what you may be going through mentally or even physically.

Maybe the main cause of a lot of your worries is the unknown answers to what will happen to your sibling; scared for them and scared for their future.

Maybe you don't want to concern your parents with the thoughts that are hidden away in your head, so you try to find other ways to figure it out independently out of respect for your sibling's complex needs and your parents' already overflowing plates. Maybe your parents are close to emotionally collapsing and you don't want to see them fall apart even more, especially if you could be the reason they finally break.

When I was in grade seven, at the age of thirteen, my mental health took a turn for the worst. It was terrifying as a child, feeling as if my mind was taken over by my body, dragging it by a leash and compelling it to do restless repetitions to alleviate my anxieties.

I would tap my feet four times before I got into my bed, I would touch the corners of the railings before going down the steps to our basement, and when I read my books, I couldn't help but re-read the sentences multiple times before I felt satisfied to finish and put it down. I would wash my hands excessively until they were so dry that they were beet red and covered with massive cracks. Worst of all, when my anxiety was so unmanageable, I would take my clothes off and put them back on multiple times because of the unease and uncomfortableness I felt in my own body.

It felt like my behaviour began to add onto the worries both of my parents already had. They wanted to help me get over these anxious thoughts that I was trapped in, but in all honesty, it was not just something I could've gotten over and gotten rid of so easily over night. People misunderstand when they don't experience it firsthand, they just assume you can just let go of the intrusive thoughts - like it's that easy.

As I became a young adult and my overall awareness of self heightened, I recognized that my anxieties went away once I became truly happy with where I was in my life. I will admit, before I found techniques to help me cope with my mental health and my OCD, I needed to go through some of the most embarrassing experiences that have ever happened to me.

I was in the parking lot at the golf course driving range on this one particular afternoon, when someone watched me have an extreme OCD episode. I began tapping my feet extremely fast for what felt like four rounds of counting to six, on the gravel parking lot out of the door of my vehicle before hopping into my car and heading home after a golf session; I was sixteen. I looked up at the surrounding cars that filled the parking lot, and I set eyes on a person staring at me from across the parking lot. He looked at me with shock written all over his face, probably wondering what the heck was wrong with me. But he had no idea how much I was struggling to even be out of the house, let alone of my own bedroom for that matter, and how much effort it took me to calm myself down in that particular moment.

In the article, Advice from Siblings Of Special Needs written by Alyson Kruegar, she stated that, "As the sibling, we have a difficult time feeling like we can express our feelings to our family or the ones closest to us. There's this fear in the back of our minds that what we want to complain about or question, could be so small and trivial compared to what our parents are going through with your sibling, and we feel we could be asking for too much during that time".

Having a mental illness is real. It's emotional, traumatic, unhealthy, and sometimes even life-threatening ... and is a very dark time.

Maybe the reason you are reading this book right now is because you are seeking answers, or for a way to connect with others in our community so you can finally feel 'normal'. Or maybe this book will be the resource you needed to feel heard and relatable.

Remember there is light after every storm, and once you get there you will find your true happiness. Live life with patience and love. When I accepted that when things didn't go as I planned or when I ran into difficult situations, I always tried to find a way out of the darkness, and some how I learned and grew, evolving from those moments.

We, as the siblings, were designed to have a greater outlook on life. We have been taught empathy from a very young age, and to be grateful for health, happiness, and most importantly, for our family's loving bond.

Being their sibling highlights all of these gifts that makes us so amazingly different, it's what makes us so incredibly special.

"*Wanting to be someone else*

Is a waste of the

person you are."

-Marilyn Monroe

YOUR PARENTS' SADNESS AND FEAR IS NEVER TRULY HIDDEN FROM THE SIB; SHARE IT, EXPLAIN IT, AND HEAL AS A FAMILY (OTHERWISE, WE BOTH GO THROUGH THIS ALONE

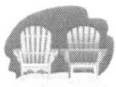

Your parents leave to bring your special needs sibling to a routine doctor's appointment, only to notice when they returned home, their whole presence changed. They're anxious, pacing down the hallways in your house, not speaking a word to anyone. Their overwhelmed emotions seep into every room of the house, and the air is so heavy it's suffocating you. Their faces are almost stained by their tears, from which you can only imagine was a never-ending cry during the car ride home.

Although, your parents try extremely hard to hide their emotions from you (the sibling) as if nothing had happened, you can't help but feel what they're going through. You sense its presence; the unsettling feeling that something terribly wrong is about to happen. All the energy soaks in like a sponge from their unexpected and uncontrollable emotions and stresses that you have now adopted as well, as if they now were your own fears.

You begin to worry because you feel their sadness and you don't know why they feel the way they do. You start to wonder if something was terribly wrong with your sibling; maybe they're not okay. Could they be sick?

Questions continue to swarm in your head, fighting for answers like a bunch of seagulls squawking and wrestling for food scraps. Thinking the unimaginable, what is going to happen to my sibling? How long do I have with them?

As I matured, I realized that I never took into consideration everything that my parents had done for my sister and me, what they had sacrificed for us, and what they were personally going through as parents. I only thought about myself, how being in a family with a special needs child impacted me and how I lost myself along the way; trying to figure out how to understand this life and how to be a sibling to my sister who was differently abled.

On the other hand, my mother tried her hardest to hide her struggles behind closed doors around my sister and me. For many years, after she'd put both my sister and me to bed at night, she couldn't help but bawl her eyes out from exhaustion, feeling so alone and fearing she was failing us. During the process of writing this book and through many conversations with my mother about this, I regret not being there for her and for not realizing how alone she really felt.

"The best is yet to come."

-Frank Sinatra

MY DEPARTING MESSAGE TO ALL THOSE SPECIAL NEEDS SIBS

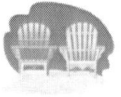

In the process of writing this book, I heard a lot of, "I didn't really think about you and your perspective as being the sibling". I've shared chapters from my book with my grandparents and I witnessed their facial expressions change immediately once they heard what I went through as a child. And my mother cried as I told her the truth of how stuck and lonely I felt; unsure of what side of the path I should have taken, and where was I going.

One morning, my mother and I met my publisher, Dawn, at a café; we were there to discuss a game plan for my book. Dawn mentioned, "It seems like after listening to you that you feel like the sibling doesn't really belong anywhere. It's as if they're just floating," I remember her saying.

And she was kind of right. I always felt stuck searching for a place, looking for the people who I could relate to, a place where I could settle in and feel like I could be my authentic self without feeling so different than everyone else or forgotten by others.

One day, my mother said to me, "After reading your book and doing some thinking, about how you may have felt as the sibling, it dawned on me that maybe you felt like you never really had both your feet planted anywhere. You had one foot in the world of disability, while the other was trying to step into the world with everyone else. It must have felt like you really couldn't be stable in either world, like you never really truly felt like you belonged, because you aren't separate from each side- you are built from both."

The truth is, I haven't had both of my feet planted anywhere. "Maybe the sibling is meant to be the bridge between these two worlds, bringing them together", my mother added. I never thought about it this way.

I felt sad facing this realization. For so long I've been struggling to find a home within these two worlds. Feeling like no one understood me, no one understood my family, and no one understood my life because it was so different from their own. When I attempted planting my feet into one world, it was only a matter of time until I felt I needed out because it didn't make sense to stay. It's difficult to be your authentic self when everyone wants you to be the same as them. So, I altered who I was, I hid parts of myself, and because of this, I never actually felt whole. The question was, how was I supposed to plant both feet in my two entirely different worlds simultaneously, without feeling I was living two separate lives- being two different versions of myself all the time. You can't, you lose yourself.

SIB: Standing In Between

Standing in what at times feels like the invisible and misunderstood realms that reside in the shadows of our siblings -

somewhere between the world of disability and the busyness and carelessness of the rest of humanity.

Perhaps we (the siblings) are placed here for a greater purpose, for a unique opportunity to be the bridge for our two worlds to finally meet; to finally be understood and embraced. Once this happens, an uplifting evolution might take place within our society. And the gift of empathy received by this union through God's love, may teach humanity how to be kinder.

We, the SIBS, collectively can unite and stand strongly and proudly with courage to use our gifts to finally bridge our two worlds together.

Perhaps we are the bridge, created to witness two worlds that rarely coexist. And because we don't feel truly the same as anyone on either side, we view each world from the shadows; not sure where we really belong as we are the product of both worlds, and so we are waiting for the two to collide and merge into one.

12 Things to Always Remember:

1)   *The past can't be changed.*

2)   *Opinions don't define your reality.*

3)   *Everyone's journey is different.*

4)   *Judgments are not about you.*

5)   *Overthinking will lead to sadness.*

6)   *Happiness is found within.*

7)   *Your thoughts affect your mood.*

8)   *Smiles are contagious.*

9)   *Kindness is free.*

10)   *Its okay to let go and move on.*

11)   *What goes around, comes around.*

12)   *Things always get better with time.*

-The Mind Journal

ACKNOWLEDGEMENTS

To my parents, who never failed to give us their unconditional love, support, and encouragement no matter what. Even when they were struggling, they continued to give my sister and me a life full of laughter and excitement. Always trying to make sure I was living a life full of opportunities and experiences and most importantly, for making sure that I was never forgotten.

To my sister: I am so grateful to have you in my life. I want to dedicate this book to you in hopes that people will understand, see, and hear you more clearly. Thank you for loving me every single day. You are my greatest gift; you will forever have my heart.

To Dawn, my publisher, my new writing friend who saw the potential in me and for this book that I have written. Thank you for your encouragement, support and for your creative mind.

And thank you, Mom, for your writing contributions and for working alongside Dawn and me, throughout the edit and revision process. Thank you for noticing when I was holding back, afraid to hurt your feelings and for giving me the permission to share my story, encouraging me to remember the importance of speaking in the most authentic and raw way, knowing it's possible that sharing the struggles we went through may help others.

I would also like to thank my Beta Readers (Julie Hanson, Deb Brooks, Deb McFarlane, Sharon Goss, Chris E, Michelle Van Manen, Marylin Dalton, and my grandmothers), and also Michelle Vine, Neil Sharp and Dr. Dan Dalton for all your contributions, support and encouragement as I went through this vulnerable and very personal process. I am forever grateful for each and everyone of you for giving me a safe space and allowing me to share my story for the first time with you all.

ABOUT THE AUTHOR

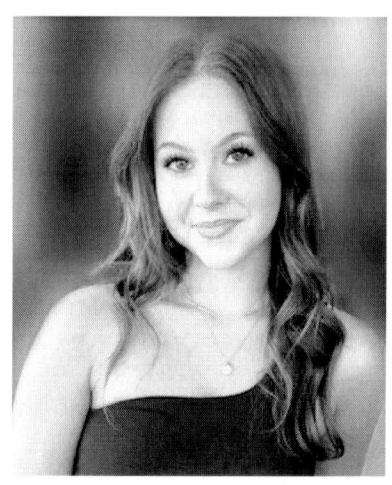

Kylainah Zacharczuk lives in Southwestern Ontario with her Golden Doodle, Lenny. She is an avid golfer, has a love for reading fantasy novels, enjoys immersing herself in yoga and meditation practices and has a current obsession with Strawberry Acai drinks from Starbucks.

RESOURCES FOR THE SIBS

Books

• The Sibling Slam Book: What it's really like to have a brother or sister with Special Needs.
Written by: Donald J. Meyer

• Thicker Than Water: Essays by Adult Siblings of people with Disabilities
Written by: Don Meyer

• Sibshops: Workshops for Siblings of Children with Special Needs (revised edition)
 Written by: Don Meyer M.Ed. and Patricia Vadasy Ph.D.

• Views from our Shoes: Growing up with a brother or sister with Special Needs.
Written by: Donald J. Meyer and Cary Pillo

• Everybody is different: A book for young people who have brothers or sisters with Autism.
Written by: Fiona Bleach

• The Siblings Survival Guide: Indispensable Information for brothers and sisters of Adults with Disabilities
Written by: Don Meyer and Emily Holl

• Out of my Mind, written by: Sharon M. Draper

- Inspiring Stories About Diversity: Empowering Tales To Teach Kids Empathy, Cultivate Kindness, Celebrate Differences and Encourage Acceptance That All Children Belong.
Written by: Lily Nicolai

- We All Belong: A Children's Book About Diversity, Race and Empathy.
Written by: Nathalie Goss, Alex Goss, and Goss Castle

- SibKits. (The SibKits ABI is a booklet filled with tools and guides for brother and sisters of children who have a disability)
Written by: Holland Bloorview- Kids Rehabilitation Hospital

Networks and Websites

- Sibling Support: www.siblingsupport.org

- https://hollandbloorview.ca/services/programs-services/sibling-support-program

YouTube Videos: What is Special Needs

- Children with Special Needs Video (Jason I am)

- OHEL 44th Annual Gala Nov 2013 Video - Siblings: Unspoken challenges, unrelating love

YouTube Videos: Mental Health

• Anna Freud National Centre for Children and Families - CARE - A Cognitive Whiteboard Animation

• Let's Talk About Mental Illness- Kids Mental Health Video by NAMI Wisconsin

RESOURCES FOR THE PARENT

Websites

- (Sibs) For brothers and sisters of disabled children and adults: www.sibs.org.uk
- 2.The Dos and Don'ts of Supporting Someone with Mental Illness, written by: The Providence Center
- https://www.providencecenter.org>news>the-dos-and ...
- Helping a Loved One Cope with Mental Illness.
- Written by: American Psychiatric Association
- www.psychiatry.org/patients-families/helping-a-loved-one-cope-with-mental-illness

- American Psychological Association (APA) How to Cope One When a Loved One Has a Serious Mental Illness
- www.apa.org> topics> serious-mental-illness

Books

- *Kids Beyond Limits* written by Anat Baniel
- *Move Into Life* written by Anat Baniel

INDEX

KidsAbility (Page 14 & 15)
https://www.kidsability.ca *"KidsAbility supports children and youth from birth to age 21 to navigate the entire journey from childhood to adulthood, irrespective of diagnosis. We believe providing early and exceptional family-centred services for the wellbeing of children and youth is the most powerful way to build brighter futures."*

BioFeedback® (Page 34)
https://my.clevelandclinic.org/health/treat-ments/13354-biofeedback
On the Cleveland Clinic website, it states that, *"Biofeedback (biofeedback therapy) is an alternative medicine approach that teaches you to change the way your body functions. It's a mind-body therapy that may improve your physical and mental health"*.

NeuroFeedback® (Page 34)
•https://neuroptimal.com/store/?campaign=21723909027&keyword=neurofeedback+equipment+for+sale&network=g&gad_source=1

•https://neurvanahealth.com/naturopathic-therapies-neurofeedback/
On the Neurvana website it states that, *"Many athletes as well as business professionals use neurofeedback regularly to improve their performance by improving alertness,*

memory, focus, clarity in both written and verbal communication."

ABM® NeuroMovement® (Page 34)
https://www.anatbanielmethod.com

Anat Baniel Method® NeuroMovement® is a holistic approach to human functioning and action. It has been endorsed by leading neuroscientists including Dr Michael Merzenich (the "father" brain plasticity science), Dr Jill Bolte Taylor, Dr Norman Doidge and Dr Elizabeth Torres. Small gentle movements, with highly refined attention to subtle differences and change facilitate the adult or child client to learn to overcome limitations and create new patterns of movement, feeling and thought. To date Anat and her team of trainers have trained hundreds of ABM® NeuroMovement® practitioners who help adults and children suffering stroke and brain injury, autism, genetic disorder and undiagnosed developmental delay, aches, pains, and other limiting factors, to attain new levels of performance, vitality, and well-being.

In 2019 Anat was approached by Lloydminster Catholic School District (LCSD) in Canada with a request to bring NeuroMovement into their schools. She created the ABC (Anat Baniel Classroom) Program which continues to evolve. It had a positive impact on learning outcomes throughout the school district at a time when other schools struggled during the Covid-19 pandemic and also lead to significant decreases in student injuries and behavioral incidents. Data collected from individual children is being analyzed by Dr Elizabeth Torres of Rutgers.

"*Anat has defined the principles of neuroplasticity in practical and understandable human terms… Anat and I, along parallel lines, have thought about the principles of neuroscience translated into therapeutics. Anat is as close as any therapist I know in having the right idea. I support ABMNM, it makes good neurological sense.*"

~Dr Michael Merzenich, Emeritus Professor of Neuroscience at UCSF, Member of the National Academy of Sciences and Winner of the 2018 Kavli Prize in Neuroscience.

Bruce Lipton (Page 35)
YouTube Video: Dr. Bruce Lipton Explains How to Reprogram Your Subconscious Mind (Fearless Soul)
www.youtube.com/watch?v=OqLT_CNTNYA

• Article: The World Health Organization- Mental Disorders (Page 126)
https://www.who.int/news-room/fact-sheets/detail/mental-disorders

• Article: Advice from Siblings of Kids with Mental Health Disorders
Written by: Alyson Kruegar (Page 130)
Website: https://childmind.org/article/advice-from-siblings-of-kids-with-mental-healthdisorders/

Psychoeducational Assessment: (Page 26 & 35)
Understanding Psychoeducational Assessments: A Guide
Hamilton Psychological Services
www.hamiltonpsych.ca> understanding>psychoeducational assessments

"A psychoeducational assessment (sometimes called a comprehensive psychological assessment), is a process designed to come to an overall picture of your strength and areas of need related to either school or work functioning. A psychoeducational assessment also is designed to make conclusions about any diagnoses that might be affecting your functioning."

What Is OCD (Page 124-127,130) National Institute of Mental health (OCD)
www.nimh.nih.gov>health>topics> obsessive-compulsive

"Obsessive-compulsive disorder (OCD) is a long-lasting disorder in which a person experiences uncontrollable and recurring thoughts (obsessions), engages in repetitive behaviours (compulsions), or both. People with OCD have time-consuming symptoms that can cause significant distress or interfere with daily life."

WHERE I FOUND MY RESEARCH

Top 5 Strategies to Cultivating your Mental Health

www.maginationpressfamily.com

www kids.britannica.com

www bucketlistjourney.net

www.trulyexperiences.com

www.positivepsychology.com

www.mantracare.org

www.mind.org.com

www.cardiac.com

*Eight things siblings of children with Special Needs struggle with-Washington Post

www.goodtherapy.org

*Advice From Siblings of Special-Needs Kids- Article written by: Alyson Krueger

www.mentalhealth-uk.org (Mental Health Conditions)

www.Sharonselby.com (Bruce Lipton)

www.Mentalhelp.net (Intellectual-disabilities)

www.en.m.wikipedia.org (Intellectual disability WIKIPEDIA)

*Pinterest- For All the Quotes

www.neurolaunch.com Understanding and Managing OCD Episodes: A Comprehensive Guide

TESTIMONIAL

Kylainah Zacharczuk

Recently, I went to a NeuroFeedback® clinic and after receiving a few sessions, I noticed great results. This treatment helps by giving the brain signals to start developing healthier patterns within the brain.

After receiving a session once a week for a month, I noticed a sense of calmness and ease. It released my constant compulsion to touch everything (my OCD triggers), a reduction in my daily anxiety, and most importantly, it helped calm my nervous system.

Manufactured by Amazon.ca
Acheson, AB